A Marathon of Changes

A Marathon of Changes

The Radical Transformation of a Baby Boomer

Jo Ann Miller

Foreword by John Glenn

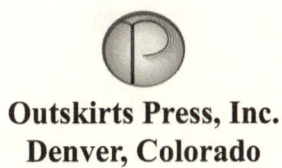

Outskirts Press, Inc.
Denver, Colorado

Grateful acknowledgement is made to April Hochstrasser, Ph.D., for permission to reprint a portion of her **The Patient's Guide to Weight Loss Surgery – Revised.**

I dedicate this book with love and great appreciation to my father, Lieutenant General (USMC) Thomas H. Miller and my mother, Ida Mai Miller. They shall forever be the wind beneath my wings.

Contents

Foreword

A tough, drastic, and life-changing decision was the choice made by Jo Ann Miller several years ago, with an emphasis on the "life changing." Such change involved her weight, or more accurately her "overweight" condition, something she grappled with unsuccessfully through most of her adult life.

This book is the story of what led to that decision and its results. If you have a major overweight problem, you may consult with your doctor and reach a different decision than described here by Jo Ann. However, the narration of what happened to her will be of major interest to you.

I have known Jo Ann since she was an infant, so I have seen the changes in her life first hand. She is a remarkable woman.

Her father-to-be and I met during Naval Aviation Flight Training in World War II, became fast friends and both became Marine pilots. By luck of the draw assignments, we were stationed together during much of our careers in the Marine Corps. We flew together during World War II and Korea and shared several common assignments here in the states. We built homes next door to each other in the Washington area. The Millers and the Glenns became one big extended family with all children in and out of both houses.

I would be surprised if you have not already peaked at the Chapter titles of this book and determined the ultimate decision of Jo Ann to culminate her "transformation."

If you do not have a weight problem, I think you will still find this an interesting account of decision making and determination.

If you do have a weight problem then you must envision what kind of life, what kind of person you wish to be five, ten or fifteen years from now and start working toward that goal. NOW! You are the only one who can make that decision.

Good luck!

John Glenn
United States Senator (retired)
Columbus, Ohio
December 2009

Preface

On February 2nd, 2005, I sat in a real estate seminar. I was bored out of my mind. So, as I had done many times before, I took out a sheet of paper and wrote down my goals for the coming year. Being the true procrastinator that I am, you will note that I waited until February until I got around to my New Year's resolutions!!!! They were:

(1) I want to feel and become healthy. I want my weight to be what it needs to be for me to feel fit. I do not want to feel self-conscious of the way I look;
(2) I want to be financially independent;
(3) I want to develop some very close trusting relationships with people;
(4) I want to learn to feel and believe good things about myself;
(5) I want to believe I deserve to have good things happen to me.

This book is dedicated to those who have had the same inspirations and problems in achieving them. I have learned through my transformation that I am very special. In no way do I mean to be boastful in my writing. My purpose is merely to encourage every reader to find this special identity within their selves. I can guarantee everyone that it is there!

Jo Ann Miller
Westport, Connecticut
November 2008

Introduction

In October of 2006, only some twenty months after I had written down my five goals at the seminar, I stood at the starting line of the Marne Corps Marathon in Washington, D.C.

My life had changed drastically. I had lost one-hundred fifty pounds and become a lean runner ready for my first attempt at the 26.2 mile marathon distance. Standing next to me at the starting area was an old college flame of decades past that had become the love of my life. He had trained me for this run every step of the way and now was going to run with me the whole distance.

In addition, I had achieved many of my goals including finding financially security, being emotionally happy and believing that I was truly special. This transformation follows my running of the marathon in direct parallels.

This was not always a smooth and easy journey. I sometimes stumbled, fell, cried, laughed and got myself up many times. It was work but well worth it. I enjoy life now in a very special and new way that I never imagined before.

As I run this marathon of life changes, enjoy the ride. I hope your journey is as much fun and brings you as much as happiness.

MILE **1**

"The thrill is overcoming your own fear."

Theodore Roosevelt

The race started at 8:00 a.m. I had been up since five a.m. after an interrupted and fidgety night's sleep. No bones about it, I was nervous!!! I was staying at my parent's house in Arlington, Virginia. It was far more convenient than a hotel and my parents were very supportive of my attempt at a marathon. They had no idea of what it took to run this race but they loved me unconditionally. The commute to the race was a marathon in itself. I took the Metro a short way but with 34,000 runners, it was like rush hour in New York City. The tension of the masses added to my stress.

I arrived early enough to stand around for a good long time. It was perhaps too long as I was getting antsy and quite irritable. I had brought some old clothes from the local Goodwill Store to keep warm. They were "throw-a-ways" that would be donated back to charity after the start of the race. It was a brilliant clear blue day but a tad chilly. It was a perfect day to run a marathon!!! I had run some long training runs in warm weather and it was no fun.

Instead of my designated spot in the back of the pack, I moved forward closer to the starting line. My number, which positioned me according to my estimated time, was concealed by my Old Navy sweatshirt. While I expected to be running at a 12 minute mile pace, I was up with the 9 minute group: a runner always wants to get to the starting line first. This was not altogether proper but made perfect sense. I sat down in the nearby curb to keep my legs fresh. My coach had forewarned me: save all the energy for the race. As I did so, my mind took me back to my early beginnings.

I was born in Hawaii before it became a state. My birth certificate proudly declares it as a territory of the United States. I remember very little of the islands for I was not there for very long. This trend of temporary domiciles would continue through much of my adolescence for I was a military "brat." I am not sure where this term originated from for I was certainly not spoiled. I was the daughter of a career Marine officer. My father was a jet pilot and later a General in charge of Marine Aviation during the Vietnam War. He was a big-time hero and I think the only pilot to fly combat missions in World War II, Korea and Vietnam. Each day my father stepped into the cockpit of his jet airplane, he looked death in the eyes. I have never seen him scared of anything. I sometimes wished I was more like him.

I grew up in the 1960's as a member of the post-war generation, so aptly called the Baby Boomers. We Boomers are grown adults now or at least some of us pretend to be. I always consider myself part of that decade of change. It was an outstanding, outrageous and totally out-of-the-box period of time. Fun was my calling card and like many others of my peer group, we lived a new lifestyle unlike any other before. This is not to say I was a "hippie" although I did believe in free love, legalized drugs and the end to a terrible war in Vietnam. I loved life and the people around me. I still do.

Looking back, my father was constantly reminding his "girls" to be watchful of what we ate. I remember exercising as a family on Saturday nights while watching "Perry Mason" and "Checkmate."

Being fit was important and being fat was frowned upon. And, as with other things in my life, I may have subconsciously rebelled against my father's commands. This is hardly an excuse for eating too much. I have learned that it is really no one's fault. It is what you do about your problems that really count.

Somebody was saying something on the microphone from the race stand. I could barely hear the introduction of the "starter." I assumed it was someone famous but really did not care at that this point. I remained nervous and apprehensive. It seemed like an endless wait and I could not wait for the speaker to stop talking and we could begin our running. I noticed, to my left, a couple snuggled together under an army blanket. He appeared to be the runner and she, dressed in street clothes, was his support staff. I wondered what kind of woman would wake up this early to watch her lover start the race.

My father married his childhood sweetheart. They met as fellow toddlers growing up in the state of Texas. They remain married today, some sixty plus years later. My parents have always been very loving parents and devoted to their children. "Pop" was an ace pilot. He set a speed record in the Phantom jet in 1962. He was not the stereotypical Marine officer. Pop was never mean or a strict disciplinarian. He loved God, his country and his family. Pop always found time to play with his three kids: my older brother Donald, my sister Jacque, and me.

My mother was beautiful and full of "fun". That word describes her to a tee. She was a housewife and married to a career military officer, which was no easy task. She was always busy coordinating events on base for the Marine families. These are the responsibilities of an officer's wife and my mother performed them exceptionally well. She also found time to write a children's book and edit the base newsletter. This may have been my inspiration to write this book

Our house was the gathering place for the neighborhood, wherever we lived. It included many of our extended military family but also many from the local area, wherever we worked. Our home was a happy place with lots of love and excitement. It was a good place to grow up even if our home base was constantly changing.

Marine pilots are usually stationed on the West or East coast, where the aviation bases are located. So we crossed this country many times as my father was transferred from California, to Rhode Island, to Virginia, back to California and so forth. We moved every two to three years. To me, that meant saying goodbye to many friends. There was never a debate about it. This was life as a military child. It was hard not to resent having to move away from my school and friends. But life went on. My mother always set the tone and tried to make each move an adventure. And also, there is no second guessing the decisions of United States Marine Corps. You did it and tried to smile. There was never a debate about one of us children staying behind. There were no options discussed. Never explain, never complain was the military disciplinary mantra.

There is a common bond between Marine families. It is not really a "misery loves company" type of thing but more of an unspoken unity among people with similar backgrounds and life-styles. All of us were very positive, even us kids. Our fathers were strong-minded individuals who loved their country and their jobs. And in most cases, they were married to very devoted wives. As a result, even if you wanted to complain, there really wasn't anyone who would listen.

Instead, you made the best of it. You endured. I was a good "soldier" in the earlier years but I would change my attitude toward authority when I became a teenager, challenging many things and asking the question "why" to both my parents. I wasn't really a rebel although I may have thought of myself as one. I even flunked my first attempt at my driver's license because I had an "attitude." As you might imagine, this didn't play very well in a Marine household.

There must have been a thousand Marines at the starting line. When the inaudible speaker stopped talking, there was a murmur among the huge crowd and then a huge BOOM arose from the cannons being shot. I was startled for it came as a complete surprise to me. There were just too many people to see what was going on up front.

Shortly thereafter, we were off. Walking! I thought we should be running although I had no idea what my hurry was? I was reassured that there was just too many people jammed into a small two-lane street to allow everyone room to run. I remained patient. Patience has never been my strong suit but, again, there was not much I could do about it. It took about five minutes to get to the actual starting line. I wore a computer chip that would gauge my exact time so I was not worried about that aspect of the run. All I wanted to do was run! I had taken the week off before the race to rest. My body was used to running and the layoff added to my nervousness and anticipation. Finally we began to jog slowly and the masses were like cattle being led to slaughter, not a cheery analogy. I could feel my heart beating quickly. I was ready and the race was beginning, however slowly. The course took us back toward the center of Arlington and my mind returned to years past.

When I was in junior high school, my father was stationed in Washington, D.C. He was moving up the chain of command quickly. His notoriety for setting the speed record had catapulted his career and he proved to be a natural leader. He was headed toward becoming a flag officer. In the Marines that means General. So my parents, with the security of his success, decided to build a house in Arlington, Virginia, where they still live today.

Next door to us at the time lived the John Glenn family. The famous astronaut had gone to flight school with my father and they had served together in World War II and Korea. They were as close as brothers and had made a promise to watch out for each other's families in case anything happened to the other. So the Glenns and Millers became neighbors when my father and "Uncle Johnny" decided to buy two lots next to each other across the street from Williamsburg Middle School in Arlington. The two families were inseparable growing up. My brother, Don, was best friends with Dave Glenn. My sister Jacque and I were very close with Lyn Glenn. I have enjoyed this extended family relationship with the Glenns my entire life. "Uncle" Johnny and "Aunt Annie" are wonderful people and I cherish our relationship together.

We would leave Arlington for California when I was starting high school. My parents decided to keep the house and rent it out when my father was stationed elsewhere. It really became my home away from home and a cheerful reminder that we had roots somewhere. It was very important to me that we kept that home and I still love that house and its memories.

The crowds had broken up by the half mile point. I felt better. I was somewhat aerobic by now, meaning I was breathing easy. It takes the resting body some time to get its oxygen level up from running and once oxygenated, your heart slows and settles your nerves. I saw the mile 1 marker and the clock read 9:12 minutes in large digital numbers. This was much too fast and I slowed down. It is a mistake to believe that if you haven't trained at a certain pace, you will be able to run faster during a race. Your body really gets used to a routine and if you deviate from that routine, your body tends to rebel. I had been forewarned that this might happen because the runner is well rested and geared up for doing well, the tendency is to go out to fast and pay for it later in the race.

At the mile mark there was also evidence of an accident. At the start, we runners had heard that one of the lead runners had suffered a heart attack right at the beginning of the race. This was the reason why we had waited so long at the start. An ambulance remained at the site with two paramedics, both looking deeply concerned. There was a lot of medical equipment spread across the grass to the side of the race route. I said a quick prayer for the runner's life.

It was in California, in 1962, when tragedy struck our family. My brother died from injuries he received in a motorcycle accident. He was only nineteen years old. It was devastating to all of us. Don was the oldest and only son. He had always watched ever so closely over his two younger sisters and all three of us were great friends, even hanging out together. My sorrow still remains indescribable. I miss Don. His death brought our family closer together and my parents somehow got through it with their strong religious beliefs. It wasn't easy but we were strong.

I never received any counseling after the death of my brother. In retrospect, perhaps, I needed it but this was not the Marine way. You kept your emotions within and remained positive. My parents encouraged this and it was in tune with their deep religious beliefs. I heard often that "God needed Donny in heaven." I never understood this deep faith or the need to merely internalize one's grief. I wanted to cry out. I was angry that my brother had been taken from us.

As I continued to run strong, I saw the first water station and grabbed an orange and cup of water. I knew it was going to be a long day.

MILE **2**

The second mile of the race was straight uphill. It was really the only incline on the course and I didn't much enjoy it. I am a flatlander. I like things flat and I like to run on flat land. Hills are for goats and skiers. As I expended more energy than normal, I could still feel the extra adrenaline in my spirit. The time off helped with this but I was also getting pumped on finishing my first marathon.

The crowds were huge at this point of the race. They were three deep in some places of the hill and turnaround at the top of this "mountain". I had chosen a very red shirt with a Marine Corps emblem, a gift from a friend, to wear this day. It was sort of like Tiger Woods wearing red on Sunday but it was also the Marine colors. I had also embossed the word "Brat" just above the emblem. The great crowds picked up on the shirt, as they did many other runners with identifiable names on their apparel. They yelled out "Go Brat" in unison and I loved it. I smiled, ran faster and waved to the well wishers. This was fun!

As we turned the corner at the top of this monstrous and seemingly endless hill, I saw a runner with a Penn State shirt to my left. My mind quickly returned to my past. In 1965, Mom, Dad and I moved to Carlisle, Pennsylvania at the end of my sophomore year in high school. Jacque went off to college. I really loved California and still sometimes think of myself as that surfing girl in a bikini on the beach. It was a wonderful place to be young.

My father was sent to the Army War College in Carlisle. It was a nice small knit community and I fit in well with the military kids, the "posties" as well as the local "townies" at the high school. I played volleyball and ran cross country. I dated the Student Body President. Life was good. I loved my junior year. It was a time of self-recovery from my brother's death and a period of great fun and joy.

Unfortunately, my father was transferred back to the Washington, D.C. area for my senior year. I attended Yorktown High School in Arlington, famous for its alumnae, Kati Couric. I hated my senior year and got a real attitude about life. I missed my old high school and decided not to make many friends. I was going off to college in a year and didn't feel the necessity of socializing. I felt that it was a waste of time. It was really the first time I became resentful of my military background. I really wanted to stay in Carlisle and have fun but the damn Marine Corps had plans for my father. I was not a happy solider. I gave true meaning to the word military "brat." You can imagine how much fun I was for my parents!

During this time, I also started to mature as a young woman. My bust and butt took shape. I think the word is robust. I like voluptuous better. I do know that I was beginning to put on weight.I had always been very active as a kid and teenager. I loved sports and was very much the tomboy growing up with some ballet background as well. My parents were athletic as well. They taught me golf, tennis, skiing and surfing. While there were not the opportunities for women in organized athletics as there are now, I kept very active in sports. I ran before it really became popular. I remember running in eighth grade, in the early sixties. I loved to run. Later in my twenties, I once ran twenty miles to the George Washington Bridge in New York City from my apartment in New Jersey. It was a beautiful day and seemed like a fun thing to do. A tad crazy maybe but I always liked a good challenge. Life was meant to be fun for me and being active was purest form of enjoyment. I kept very active and like my mother was often in constant motion. I am very much my mother's daughter.

Weight was never an issue back then for me. I can't remember being concerned about it and I know I wasn't ever afraid to be seen in a bathing suit. I ate a balanced diet and my mother was a great cook. She also liked to bake great desserts but was very strict on their consumption. Sugar was limited. Junk food just did not exist in my life. The younger reader may find that hard to believe but there was just not a Burger King or MacDonald's on every block back then.

I did start to put on weight my senior year in high school. I was sort of down about leaving Carlisle for Virginia. Perhaps this may have had a part in the increase in weight. I have never analyzed whether or not the combination of the anxiety and my developing body may have caused me to rely on food as an emotional lift. It may well have been the reason but like many teenagers, I didn't give it much thought.

MILE **3**

"If you remember the 1960's, you probably didn't live them."

Tom Hayden

There was no water at the mile three marker. It was getting warm and I knew I needed to stay hydrated. They did provide some oranges and I grabbed one along with a stick of Vaseline. I had learned from my long training runs that I tend to chafe along my inner thigh. I stopped for a minute and applied it to my crotch area. Runners are not real bashful about their bodies. Up on the hill to my right were a bunch of guys going to the bathroom. They didn't bother to hide behind a tree. There was a woman up there too. She did squat behind a tree and it appeared that she carried her own toilet paper. Maybe she was a Marine? Semper Fi lady! There was a bunch of Georgetown students just beyond the mile marker. They were making a lot of noise and screamed "Brat!" when I went by. I waved heartily and remembered my days back in college.

My college of choice was Upsala College in East Orange, New Jersey. My sister was already attending there and I had visited the campus several times. Jacque and I were hardly similar in personalities but it seemed like a natural selection. I liked the school. It was small with only 1,500 students and also close to New York City where one could escape the college life. So in 1967, I started school and was an art major. Don't ask me why? I am not sure to this day. But I loved to paint and sculpt and that was part of the major. Life was good at Upsala and I still have fond memories of my time there.

I dated a lot in college. I was a cheerleader and was attracted to some of the athletes. I dated one blond curly-haired soccer player, named Carl, but, after a super date, I dumped him. Much more on him later. In my junior year, I met my future husband, Richie. He was a smart sexy guy from a very Italian family. We worked in the student council and the college theatre together. After dating for a good while, we started living together late in my junior year. While it was the 1970's and the sexual revolution was in full bloom, I never told my father. Do you blame me?

I also became very active in protesting the Vietnam War. Despite my military background, I hated the War. It just made no sense to me. Richie and I helped organize transportation to the "March on Washington" in the spring of 1970 following the Kent State shootings. Hundreds of thousands attended that protest rally. As you can imagine, my father was not pleased with my anti-war feelings and actions. On one visit home, with my long hair flowing in curls and wearing army surplus apparel, my father and I got in a real verbal fight over the war. Years later he admitted that he was not all that enthused with the direction of the military at that time but during that visit, we got in a screaming match. This, of course, didn't accomplish much but I think I held my ground. We agreed to disagree which was very adult of me. And like most things with a family, we got over it.

"Life itself is the proper binge."

Julia Child

At this stage of the race, I was feeling great. The jitters were gone as well as the cobwebs from running for a full week before the race. I wasn't exactly a race horse but my body had gotten used to run. The human body is made for running. Our arms pull our legs, fueled by our core area. The only problem is that we were not made to run on hard surfaces. We were made to run on dirt or grass. That is one reason that is rash of knee and hip injuries these days.

By mile four, I was aerobic and my body was fully oxygenated. The theory of aerobics was developed by Dr. Kenneth Cooper back in the 1960's for the Air Force. To determine your aerobic heart rate, you subtract your age from the number 220 and multiply it by 75%. In my case, my aerobic heart rate is 132. When you are aerobic, your heart is working at its best and the heart muscle is being strengthened. A good test is whether you can run and have a conversation at the same time. In this state, you are not breathing hard and running actually is very enjoyable. I was at this point now. It is a great feeling and it allows your mind to wander to points often nicknamed the "runner's high."

We swung around another corner and the beauty of a long line of runners guarded by numerous Marines was really a sight to be seen. There were police holding back traffic. I wondered if they were trying to get to work. If they were, it was going to be a long wait. Plus, it was Sunday. Who was working on this day of rest? I certainly was!!!

After graduating college in 1971, I found a job in retailing with a large department store chain. For those who do not know, retailing involves the purchasing and sales of items to the consumer. It is not an easy job and to be good at it, one needs to be good with numbers and have an ability to juggle several things at once. I had always liked to work. I had many jobs in high school and worked throughout college. It was not really the money, although I liked the independence money gave me, but more the fact that work kept me busy. I hate to be bored and I have always been high energy. I am not sure whether my parents instilled in me a sense of urgency to get things done but I don't like to sit idle. Work became my passion.

My first job in retailing was at Bambergers in Newark, New Jersey. Bambergers was a division of Macy's, the huge department store based in New York City. At Bambergers, we were very proud of being the most profitable department store in the country. I started work in the summer of 1971, right after graduation from Upsala. I was placed in the executive training squad. Within a month, all trainees were assigned to a permanent position. I was made an assistant buyer of the "Little Girls" sportswear department where I helped select merchandise for the stores and distribute them to the various stores based on selling trends in each store. My job involved evaluating sales and communicating with the department managers.

I would travel to the New York market one or two times a week. It was a demanding schedule and I worked twelve hours a day six days a week. Retailing is fast paced. If you spend too much time over-analyzing the numbers, you could miss out on maximizing sales. It is a balancing act really and sometimes you just have to go with your gut and your experience.

I was promoted to department manager of men's wear in one of Bamberger's largest stores. I was responsible for managing the sales force and the presentation of the merchandise. This was really a great job for me. I was always on the move and I really enjoyed the interaction with the customers and the buying line. I received a second promotion to Group Manager, which was really the boss of department managers. My rise to this position was really too fast and I found that I was too young for the job. I realized that not everyone liked to work as hard or long as I did. I had to learn to help others have the same job satisfaction. I floundered for awhile but I eventually got the knack of it.

Within two years, I was promoted to a full fledged "buyer." Now I got to choose what went on the sales floor. I traveled to Japan and Hong Kong twice a year. Eventually I would get promoted to buyer of "Designer Sportswear" and travel around the world. I loved it. I always focus better when I am working and staying in constant motion. Books put me to sleep. In college, I went to every class and took notes. I survived because I listened to the lectures. If I had relied on just reading the text, I would have been lost. Also, I found that I worked very well face to face. My Aunt Lucy, my mother's sister, calls me a natural salesperson. I am not sure about that but I like people and I enjoy interacting with them. I am usually upbeat and positive. I think that is important to success in life. I look for the best in people. Most times, if you look hard enough, you find the good in everyone.

"Inside every older individual is a younger person wondering what the hell happened?"

Cora Harvey Armstrong

After spending the first stage of the race course in my native Arlington, we were now heading back to the capitol. We approached the Key Bridge and I could see Georgetown University in the background. I was feeling strong, the crowds were great and I was truly enjoying myself. At this juncture, I felt it was a great idea to train and run a marathon. I also realized that I had a long way to go. On the corner of the bridge in a slight gap of no spectators, I noticed a Marine in his dress blues. It was a rare sight to see as most of the volunteer Marines wore their fatigues. He was a very large and resembled someone in my past. His appearance caught my breath and took me back to a horrendous incident in my life.

The week after Thanksgiving, 1972, I was on "cloud nine" and very happy. I had just become engaged to Richie and work was going extremely well. Yet my euphoria was not to last and my strong belief in the good of people was severely tested. I was attacked and raped in the parking lot of my apartment complex in New Jersey. He was a big man who approached me when I got out of my Volkswagen and forcefully took me in the back seat of my own car. The rapist approached me in the parking lot. He was carrying a knife and a gun. I was petrified. He drove my car to another parking area nearby and then raped me in the back seat. When he was finished, he told me to wait thirty minutes. I waited five and then drove like a bat out of hell to my own place. I was barefoot in the freezing cold and Richie was waiting for me. I was hysterical. The police were called and arrived quickly. They took me to the hospital to make sure I was okay and to collect evidence. I can not describe the anger at the violation of my body, mind and dignity I felt toward this man. I was deeply humiliated and scared.

The rapist, who ironically was an ex-Marine, was eventually apprehended and jailed. My future husband was enraged and true to his Italian heritage, ashamed that he had not protected me better. I think I was so busy being concerned about his anger that I often forgot my own emotions. Maybe this was good? I am not sure to this day how I was supposed to act. Perhaps I needed counseling? It was approximately ten years after the loss of my brother. I think I was wondering if there was a reason why bad things were happening to me? While, I did not dwell on them, these thoughts lingered in the back of my mind. Needless to say, it was a difficult period for Richie and me.

I told very few people about the rape. There remains a stigma attached to this kind of crime. Too many, I think, blame the woman in somehow provoking the man into committing this type of horrific crime. This is terribly wrong. It certainly was not true in my case and I doubt with most other women. At the time, I decided to let it go emotionally. I did press charges and saw justice done giving me a small sense of redemption. I have not dwelled on this period in my life. I am not that kind of person. In a way, I feel lucky just to be alive after such a scary incident but I will take this sexual violation to my grave.

I had a moment of panic when I saw the Marine in his dress blues who resembled my rapist but it was only fleeting. This is one extraordinary aspect of running. It is a great stress reliever. Running makes you feel alive. It allows your mind to freely search through your past, sort through ideas and feel totally focused while you get the physical benefits of the exercise. Previously, I had only experienced this kind of satisfaction and relaxation through my work. That may sound crazy but work was very soothing to my soul.

Work became my life in the 1970's. I quickly climbed the corporate ladder. I was good at being a retail buyer. I was good with figures and could make quick decisions. I worked all the time. Nights, weekends and even holidays. I liked the fast pace of the retail world. Everyone wore nice clothes and in some ways, the job was glamorous. In other ways, it was demanding and exhausting. It took its toll on Richie's and my relationship. At his insistence, we married shortly after the rape incident. Richie wanted to protect me but I needed my freedom. Plus, Richie was working at night as a reporter and I worked during much of the day. We hardly saw each other. The demands of employment and the emotional baggage of the rape destroyed the marriage. We divorced within two years of our wedding.

I lived alone a short distance from New York City. I never thought anything about living by myself in a big city. The military background helped me with that sense of independence. We "brats" learned early that you were on your own in this life. I commuted to the Big Apple each day. I really liked my life. The money was great and I got to travel extensively.

My social life was just okay. At twenty-seven years of age, I lived with a very good looking guy for a time. He was almost beautiful. He turned the heads of women and men when we took walks in the city. But he liked drugs and that didn't jive with my idea of a good time. I then fell in love with a co-worker, a married man from Atlanta. We spent many fun times together while traveling. The relationship allowed me the privacy of my own life in New York and romance when traveling for work. But within a year, he was killed in an automobile accident. I was devastated. He was truly a caring man and turned me on to many new adventures. I mourned his death for a very long time.

Once again, work brought me back to reality. Since I was not having much luck with men or seemingly jinxed with the loves of my life, I just worked harder. I traveled to Europe and the Far East on business many times. On a trip to Milan, Italy, my plane was hit by lightening. The plane turned sideways and the pilot pulled out, nearly hitting some trees. It took four attempts to finally land. Another time, I was headed to Sri Lanka from Singapore. On our way, the captain announced that there had been a bombing at the airport in Sri Lanka. We landed but when I departed the plane, I saw all sorts of debris on the runway. A plane, split in half and the target of the bombing, sat directly across from where I stood. As I grew older, the retail business and its ever challenging demands were wearing on me.

MILE **6**

"Food is like sex: when you abstain even the worst stuff begins to look good."

Beth McCallister

We runners crossed the Key Bridge and entered the northwest section of the capitol known as Georgetown. Here lived the college kids from the nearby university and they were large in number and loud. Big time loud! They seemed to be having a good time as spectators but surely they did not know their great effect on the runners. For those who are "outwardly motivated" like myself, the cheers from the crowd are a tremendous lift. For those who watch a marathon, remember you do make a big difference even though the runners may be too dang tired to acknowledge it. And by the way, thank you!

Our pace was somewhat slower now. The sun was getting hot and I geared down to make sure I was not overdoing it. There was a long way to go. Patience is a key to the marathon. Those who go out too fast and do not pace themselves will not make it to the finish line. Your body gets used to a certain speed and may rebel if you alter your rhythm. Sometimes life is like this but sometimes change is good.

After ten years of working in the Northeast, I took a job in Kansas City. I was now thirty-five years old and I figured a change in scenery would do me good. Plus the salary was fantastic. The Midwestern culture was certainly different but I have found that people are much the same wherever you go. They reminded me of my extended military family: very caring but guarded individuals, conservative people with defined values. I was able to buy my first house while working in Kansas. It was a new and exciting time for me. I remained active but my weight started to escalate. For the first time in my life, I really considered myself heavy. I hid it very well with designer clothes but it was an uncomfortable feeling. I certainly did not like it. I began to try various ways of losing weight. I lost sixty pounds after seeing a hypnotist and then kept it off by going to a local diet center. I was always very successful with dieting. I lost seventy pounds again on the same plan several months later. However, I just could not keep it off. It usually would reappear within six-to-eight months.

I walked nearly every day and felt good but the weight inched itself back in time. I loved salty food. Sugar was never my problem but if a bag of chips or popcorn was available, it would be gone. Quickly! I never really binged on food or drink during times of stress. I was happy with my success in my life. I had friends. And, while I was alone in life, I wasn't lonely. I liked my privacy but enjoyed group activities as well. So looking back, I don't think I was an emotional eater nor did I eat a lot at one sitting. But I began to realize when I got on the scale that the extra pounds were coming from someplace.

MILE **7**

"I keep trying to lose weight but it keeps finding me."

Albert Einstein

By this stage of the race, we were leaving the Georgetown area and heading toward the White House. The crowds were enormous and I felt a thrill running with this many people watching. I wondered if President Bush would be out there watching the marathon but I doubted it. He had run one marathon in 1993 in Houston and done very well but his plate was pretty full these days.

My left knee had a touch of pain. As a runner, you become constantly aware of every ache and pain that may occur in your body. It is not really being a hypochondriac but a necessity of familiarity with your body. One can usually tell if your pulse is too high or that a tendon is overused. It is another way of being totally alive. I popped another Advil. I had taken two before the race but the pain meant that they had not worked or that the knee was bad. The professionals will tell you not to take pain medicine while you are running because it will mask the pain, which is your indication that something is wrong. However, this was the race, the big day and exceptions had to be made. I had plenty of time to recover once this race was over! I carried about ten pills in a plastic bag in my pocket as well as some throat lozenges as well for any dryness in my throat and some honey for energy. Each runner is different but you have to find out what works for you.

In 1984, I moved back to the New York area and purchased a house in Connecticut. It is probably the best thing I ever did. I loved the Northeast with its seasons and I enjoyed the suburbs. I liked the community atmosphere of the small town. I liked my neighbors. I also liked the money that I was being paid. My new job with the retail industry, while requiring much more time that I had been used to, was paying me more money than I had ever made before. My career had blossomed. I was comfortable with the workload and I knew I was good at what I did. It continued to be a busy time for me. I commuted to New York City every morning on the train. I worked long hours and then had a two hour commute home every night.

I had lost some weight in Kansas City but it came right back and I was now well over 200 pounds. My high school weight was 132 pounds so I was really obese. Even with the weight, I was never sick and my blood pressure remained low. I worked out: yoga, biking, rowing. But nothing seemed to work. I was fit and fat. Was that possible?

MILE **8**

"I am allergic to food. Every time I eat, it breaks out into fat."

Jennifer Greene Duncan.

The wind picked up along Pennsylvania Avenue and the President was no where to be seen. The cool air felt good at my back as I had begun to sweat heavily with the temperatures fast approaching 75 degrees. Hydration is a key here and I made sure I took some water at the aid station. There was water, Gatorade and oranges every two miles. You can imagine there is a lot needed for over 34,000 runners. A first sign of dehydration is cramping in a runner's leg. My right calf felt a tad sore and I reminded myself to take an extra amount of water at the Mile 10 station. At this stage of the race, I was not tired but I was certainly aware that I had been running for well over an hour and a half.

I passed by a sign for a local Bambergers and my mind left my aching body and returned to my past. At the end of the decade, I took another retailing job with Britches in the Washington, D.C. area. I was promoted to Vice-President and headed up two women's divisions specializing in "career wear" and sportswear. Now I was overseeing the buyers and they reported to me. I was close to the very top and I loved it. I did not want to sell my house in Connecticut so I commuted weekly. I would fly to Washington on Sunday night or Monday morning and return that Friday. It was a hellacious schedule to meet. I didn't mind the work, although that too had become seriously overwhelming. But the hassle of the travel was becoming too much. The retail industry needed me more than ever since money makers were in scare supply with a slumping economy, and I was making them a good profit.

I remained healthy and feeling okay. I have to thank my parents for I was blessed with great genes. My weight, however, was not good. I wore extra large designer clothes. I avoided every photo opportunity whether it was a family Christmas picture or a party get-together. I was now very aware of my size. In many ways, I was ashamed and embarrassed about my appearance. My friends didn't seem to care but I did. To keep my mind off the weight problem, I worked.

After only one year of doing this long distance commuting, I had had enough. I was exhausted, both physically and emotionally. I was also bored with retail now. There were no more challenges for me and work had become too much of a drudgery. I had been working hard for twenty years in an industry that never lets up.

In a coincidence that would change my life, a fellow commuter was married to a real estate agent in the Connecticut area. We became very good friends and she convinced me to give up my career in retail and join her in the real estate business. I did so in 1990 after close to twenty years in the retail business.

"You must be the change you wish to see in the world."

Mahatma Gandhi

We took a big corner after this mile marker and again the slow parade of runners moving in unison amazed me. Each runner had his or her own story. There are so many great stories about lives changed because of this form of exercise. For those who do not run or ballyhoo it because it is bad for your bones or is boring, don't know running. The sport is about getting to know yourself and what you are capable of doing both physically and mentally. The marathon is more a mental race. Your mind is telling you to quit: that you are too tired or hurt to continue to run. But your body can do amazing things. Therefore, you have to train your mind, as well as your body, to go the distance.

The different life as a realtor was and is fun but very demanding. The area I lived and worked in was one of the most affluent in the country. Houses sold for one million dollars and more. To attract customers that would trust my judgment was a bit scary, especially because I was starting this new career at the age of forty-one. I had been a retail buyer and now I was an agent for buyers and sellers. The job of a realtor was much different than I anticipated. Clients expect you to work whenever they don't, which means weekends, nights or at their convenience. I began to realize that I was very much the "people pleaser" and found the relationship in finding people homes very exciting and fulfilling.

I lucked out in working for a very good mentor, Wade Shavell, who took me under his wing and taught me the essentials of the housing market. There are many little tricks of the trade that are required if you are going to be successful. It is not always enough to be a good salesperson. You must know the law, construction and how to put a deal together. The retail industry provided me with a good foundation but I was in a new arena now. The challenge excited me.

Many of the buyers were looking for an investment. Some were Wall Street lions that expected to get a return on their very large expenditure in a house. But I approached it somewhat differently. I never went "house hunting" with people. Instead, I found a house and then went looking for a potential buyer, much like merchandising product in the retail business. It worked well for me and I worked hard at my new career. Once again, my work became my life and my passion. I worked constantly and don't even remember taking a day off or a vacation.

With the new career came a different work schedule. Often times, I would work at night and be off in the morning. My eating patterns changed with this new- found flexibility of work schedule. And I gained more weight. The structure of the retail industry, where you would have breakfast, lunch and dinner each day, went by the wayside. I ate when I was hungry and when I had time. This, unfortunately, was not what my body needed. Once again, however, life was good. I had a nice house in a beautiful suburban town. Many of my retail friends would come out from the city on weekends and we would party and have fun. I had a pool and tennis court on my property and my house, nicknamed "Camp Miller Time" became the focal point of enjoyment. It was much like the way I grew up with my parents and their Arlington home.

"It's not women's fault that diets don't work. It's not perversity of lack of willpower. God did this on purpose --- in her great wisdom."

Dr. Wayne Callaway

The veteran marathon runners tell you that if you are tired after ten miles in a marathon, it is going to be a very long day. It was beginning to get warm but the Advils were doing their job. My legs felt strong and the pain in my neck had disappeared. I thought about taking one more pill but thought I would wait until the half-marathon-mile marker. I was running at about a twelve minute a mile pace. This is a snail pace compared with the leaders who would cross the finish line with a sub-five minute mile average. It is incredible to think that a human can run that fast for so long. Much of it is genes but also much hard work. I was content to be in the back of the pack with the "penguins," as they are affectionately called.

As we continued to wander through the District's beautiful monuments, I thought back to when I first moved back to

Connecticut and my new neighbors. One of the nice things about the suburbs is that you actually get to know your neighbors. Mine were special. They were a brother and sister, Joey and Helen, both life-long residents of the town. They were of Hungarian descent and not only became very dear friends but surrogate parents to me. They were much older than me and I helped them with many physical things that they were unable to do for themselves. Despite my weight, I still had a lot of energy and was strong as an ox.

In turn, Joey and Helen watched over me and my newly acquired golden retrievers, Sarah and Bro. We were like one big happy family. The dogs really became my kids. I sometimes regretted choosing a career over children but the animals were a great substitute. They never talked back either! I woke early every morning and took them for a walk at the nearby school yard and then again in the evening. I loved the peace of my walks with them. They were my best friends among a stable of very caring individuals that was now my extended suburban family. I felt loved and very blessed to have added such a dimension to my life.

There were a few bumps along the road. My parents got very sick. My mother nearly died from complications arising from a misdiagnosis in the hospital. My father was stricken with cancer and had to undergo several operations. And my sister moved from a nearby town in Connecticut to a more rural setting in Massachusetts. She and I had always been very close. Although very different in many ways, she has two boys and I missed watching them grow up. The extended Miller clan in Connecticut went through some disagreements and spats as we grew older. Some moved and some moved on to different fun. My dear sweet neighbors got old and then sick. Helen was stricken with Alzheimer's and I had to devote a year off from work to help her and her brother. The dogs grew old quickly too. They passed away after my love and every known cure failed to prolong their lives. It was a tough road to maneuver at times. I remained strong with so many changes but it was not easy. The one constant through these difficult times was my weight. I remained heavy. But just as things were changing around me, I was about to make changes for myself.

"Gluttony is an emotional escape, a sign something is eating us."

Peter DeVries

At this stage of the race, the mind is fresh but the body is really beginning to feel the pounding. I have never calculated how many times my feet hit the pavement in each mile but it was a lot. Some have calculated it to be well over 1,000 times per mile. And I was beginning to feel every step forward. I have very high arches and while this may help you fit into a pair of high heels, it is not great for running. The higher the arch, the less support you have for your legs. Since my legs were tuned from "spinning", an act of simulated biking on a stationary bicycle, my main strength was in my lower half. Ideally, however, you want a strong upper body to carry you along on your journey. The elite runners are erect when they run. I noticed that I had a begun to slump over like an old woman with a bad back. This was not good and I straightened myself up and tried to run from my hips rather than my legs only. Certainly my age played a large part in my limitations as a runner as well as all things in life.

When you are fifty years old and really heavy, life is different. It was for me, at least. You smile, even laugh on occasion. You tend to enjoy the lives of others rather than yours. It is not necessarily a sad life. But it was one of trepidation and a fear of becoming sick or being the target of ridicule. Being heavy haunts you. It is an inescapable fate that has little escape.

In the 1990's, watching the years pass as I approached a half century on this earth, there was not one moment that I didn't think about losing weight. There was not a day I didn't think about changing and being thin again. It was frustrating and I just did not know what to do. I explored and tried all the diets available. I wanted desperately to return to my youthful body of years past.

My life was a series of getting things done. I was a doer. I had been successful at making money for a retail corporation and now for a real estate company. I had reaped the many benefits of such accomplishments but I did not feel fulfilled. There was something missing in my life. I felt empty inside although my life was full. I still worked hard and enjoyed many friends but my inner soul was hurting. And I knew it.

I attacked the problem the best way I knew how. I read everything about dieting and researched the best way to lose weight. I tried the Diet Center, NutriSystem, Fit For Life, Jenny Craig, The Zone, The Atkins Revolution, Weight Watchers, Overeaters Anonymous, Richard Simmons, The Cabbage Soup Diet and countless others. I went to doctors, nutritionists, shrinks, hypnotists and acupuncturists. I tried to meditate. I went to wellness programs. I was successful in losing weight on each and every program I tried. However, after several months, the unwanted pounds would just reappear. There was no apparent trigger. I still was not really an emotional eater. I continued to work out and really got into "spinning" and even became certified to teach a class. Even still, the overweight continued.

I listened to motivational gurus including Tony Robbins, Wayne Dyer, Deepak Chopra, Marianne Williams, Oprah and Doctor

Phil. The "mantras" I would put on little pieces of paper around my house become almost comical. I woke up one morning to find a note on my bathroom mirror that said, "You can do anything you put your mind to." So I went back to bed!!!

Despite these frustrations, I kept busy working and exercising. My energy remained high even with my excess weight. Along with my spinning, I played tennis and skied every chance I got. I walked the dogs each morning. I worked in my yard like a teenager. I felt good except when I looked into the mirror. So why was I so concerned with losing weight? If I were skinny would I be happier? Would I be able to do more things with even more energy? Was I being too impractical with my expectations? There were so many questions that my mind was in a tailspin.

There are no simple answers to these questions. Our culture certainly places a large emphasis on being thin and attractive. This is especially true with women or, at least, that is my perception. All celebrities appear to be in good shape (even though many smoke to avoid overeating). Fat people are looked upon as weak, lazy and unattractive (again my perception). Regardless of these thoughts, my biggest concern was that my obesity would eventually affect my health. I would suffer some kind of disability and not be able to be active. This was frightening to me.

MILE **12**

"Being menopausal can mean you are close to being a sociopath."

Erma Bombeck

Unfortunately for some runners, they were already dropping out of the race. I knew it was warm but this seemed fairly early on to quit the race. I did not like to use that word but what else do you call it? I certainly had no intention of dropping out. The race would kill me or I would finish. This may have been my Marine gene within.

I crept passed an aged runner and noticed the back of his t-shirt. It explained that he had run all twenty-nine Marine Corps Marathons. He was probably in his 70's and was moving at a snail's pace. "You okay?" I asked. "I just keep moving" was his only response. I was somehow relieved that he was feeling it too but there was a long way to go. No time to be yapping with a fellow runner. "Congrats on your achievement," I yelled. He nodded and I was on my way. I always noticed how many people were passing me or I was passing. Perhaps it is some kind of competitive thing but I did it throughout the race. I noticed now

I was going past people rather than the other way around. This made me feel good or at least better. Maybe I was stronger than I thought?

At the age of forty-six, I began to go through menopause. I went to a nutritionist and told him I was only having my period every other month. He recommended a regiment of supplements and diet. I began spinning five days a week. And once again, the pounds began to disappear. I lost seventy pounds and my period came back every month. The nutritionist told me that I had turned the clock back on my age. I told him that was great but I really didn't want my period back!

Eventually, menopause did set in and I lost my period. I also gained all the weight back. My joints began to hurt with the continuing exercise. I sprained my ankle. My feet hurt. Mentally and emotionally, I was getting more and more frustrated. I was out of control with my eating habits. Everything looked and tasted good. The menopause had slowed down my metabolism even more. My weight sky-rocketed and I really became down and out emotionally. I felt like I had no control over my body or my life.

Since going through menopause, I have read that fat cells actually help you in the transition. If there is one good thing about being fat, that would be it. The New Millennium found me obese but content with my life. The real estate market in Connecticut was booming and I was busy. I was making good money and was actually dating a good guy. It didn't last too long but it was fun while it lasted. He was an executive with General Electric and worked with two dear old friends. It was a good mix, the four of us. He liked to drink. A lot!!! Maybe I was becoming the gal who looked better after a couple of drinks? He did help me with my self-esteem. I found that being with someone was nice but not essential. I was fine alone or at least I convinced myself that I was. I was still very much the people person but I liked time alone as well. I was beginning to learn more and more about myself as I got older and also started to examine reasons why I was overweight. I knew

I was a perfectionist. I liked things in order. This was probably the principle reason why I was so frustrated with my weight. I could not control it. So my life continued, much as it had. I walked my dogs, worked, worked some more and took care of my neighbor Joey in my spare time.

On a trip home to visit my parents in Virginia, I was sitting at the computer without much to do. I casually, without a true purpose, typed in the words "weight loss surgery" on Google. The computer is great. It is like having a friend that knows all the answers without judging you on why you want to know. Just by the push of a few buttons on a computer, you have all your information. Within minutes, I was engrossed in reading about all the various medical procedures available to alter the digestion of food in the stomach. It was truly an inspiration to me.

I rarely went to the doctor, let alone the hospital. As I have explained, I am blessed with good genes. Yet, the thought of an operation to help me control my appetite, my consumption of food and eventually my weight really seemed very rational and simple. I found a website, www.obesity.com, on the computer that detailed testimonials of people who had undergone such surgeries. I found their stories very similar to mine. They were ordinary people who could not stop eating. Many stated that they had lost hundreds of pounds and the surgery had not only changed but saved their lives. There was one woman's story that I found fascinating. Her name was Bette and she described in great detail her own surgery. She had lost an incredible amount of weight and found a new life. She had been miserable before the procedure and now loved every day of her new life. I felt so elated and excited. It was like I had found a soul sister. Her experience was the same as mine and now she was wonderful. There was hope for me!! There was an answer to all my questions and a solution to all my frustrations. This surgery was it!!!

*"This bridge will only take you halfway there, to those mysteri-
ous lands you long to see."*

Shel Silverstein

Half way to the finish! Or at least just about half way for 13.1
miles was exactly half way. You laugh but one-tenth of a mile can
be the difference in finishing and not or so I had been told. The
crowds had increased in this area as we runners had become a
visitor's attraction. People who had come to see the monuments
on the Washington Mall, now were cheering us runners. Many
of the spectators were foreign, with cameras hanging from their
necks, baseball caps and souvenir sunglasses. But there is a universal language in running. Barriers are not set up by an inability
to speak the language. You see someone "busting his ass" and
you clap. This is a universal language of road racing that these
visitors certainly understood and their applause was almost thun-
derous. It certainly motivated me and my stride picked up a tad.
The half-way marker of a marathon is also a place where you
meet many friends or family. New shoes or socks are exchanged

or maybe a fresh towel to wipe your brow or a special drink or food is there for you. However, my buddies and "pit crew" were waiting for me at mile 22 in Crystal City. Still a long way to go! But I thought of it in a positive way. 13.1 miles finished. A new beginning for the next half marathon.

I sat for two hours in front of the computer during that stay with my parents when I was researching the possibility of the surgery. I am sorry to say I didn't spend much time with my parents on this trip. I was now on a mission. I became instantly focused and determined. I came back from Virginia and started to take action. It was my own beginning. By chance, one of my fellow realtors was married to a doctor who specialized in this type of surgery. Was this coincidence or my fate? I was beginning to feel so good about how things were falling into place, I was almost giddy. I was also smart enough to know that the solution to my problem was not simple. I knew it would involve a drastic overhaul of my life-style and my eating habits. The computer testimonials had taught me that.

I had always been embarrassed about my weight. Many of my buddies would later tell me that they never thought of me as that fat. We sure didn't talk about it though. Having a doctor that had some connection with my regular life made a difference to me. He was not just an outsider but completely objective about my person. He was married to a friend of mine. This was important to me. I felt safe and secure. His name was Dr. Craig Floch, a board certified gastrointestinal specialist in this type of weight-loss surgery. He is younger than I, quite handsome and has a very calm, easy manner about him. I had known him socially for some time. I liked him a lot.

There is much to learn when you are thinking about and con-templating gastric bypass surgery. You don't just make up your mind and make an appointment for the operation. There is a series of seminars I had to attend before any doctor would even consider me as a candidate for the procedure. The doctor wanted me to know the pros and cons of the surgery. This made perfect sense to me but was sort of scary. Was this dangerous? The seminars taught me that there is danger in any operation and that you had to prepare yourself for some drastic changes in the functions of your body. I listened carefully and read everything on this type of surgery. I was very focused and felt a real twinge of hope for the first time in a long while.

The seminars were led by former patients. They gave their testimonials on how the surgery had worked for them. Their before/after pictures were amazing and very impressive. The patients also spoke of their problems with the early states of preoperative diets and of gaining a positive attitude toward change. For many of these individuals, they had always been fat. They also were unfamiliar with any form of exercise. Without judging them, I felt confident that I could succeed as they had done.

A good doctor's office should take care of everything relating to the surgery. This includes the handling of all the insurance issues and the various tests that are needed to make sure that you are a good candidate for gastric bypass surgery. The nurses weigh you and determine your BMI (Body Mass Index). The BMI is very important in determining your acceptability for the surgery. By definition, BMI is determined by an individual's body weight divided by the square of their height. A BMI over 30 means that the patient is overweight, over 40 means obesity. Mine was 43. It was a reality check for me as my vital signs and blood chemistry was good. I have always had low blood pressure and my pulse was low due to all the "spinning" exercise. But doctors use the BMI index as a clear guide for who needs the surgery. The additional blood tests determine whether you are a high risk on the operating table.

My relationship with Doctor Floch was excellent because he is a very sincere gentleman. His first question to me: "Why do you want this surgery?" My answer was simple. "I wanted to lose weight"!! He asked me how I thought I had gained all the weight and wanted to know my attempts to lose it. He seemed impressed with my energy level and love for physical activity. I felt a little like a schoolgirl trying to please the teacher. I knew I wanted the surgery but would I meet the criteria?

This was just the beginning of the procedure to get approved for the surgery. Insurance companies require that one's primary doctor must write a letter explaining what benefits the patient would receive by having the operation. This is critical for insurance approval, and the cost of gastric bypass surgery runs about 20-30 thousand dollars. Therefore, insurance is usually a must. Each insurance carrier may differ and unfortunately, they are becoming far more stringent in their guidelines for approval. Many insurance companies have deemed gastric bypass as elective surgery and deny coverage. Unless it is "life threatening" your request for benefits may be denied. Generally, if a policyholder's weight endangers his or her overall health, then such an operation is considered preventative and allowed. This is obviously an ambiguous gray area, ripe for interpretation. Many carriers feel that a balanced diet and exercise can solve the problem. I don't think they fully understand the complicated issues involved, both physically and emotionally, in being obese. This trend in denial of coverage needs to be changed for the surgery certainly has helped many obese people. It helps people lead much healthier lives and in the long run saves the insurance companies money.

The process of receiving approval from not only the insurance company but the doctor includes visits to a nutritionist and a therapist. Both are necessary to make sure you are ready for the surgery. As you can see, this long process in gaining approval is no simple deal. It takes time and patience. Yet, I think it insures your readiness. Too many would-be patients are in a big hurry and looking for a quick fix. I was anxious to start my new beginning but abided by all the requirements. I religiously went to all the seminars, kept doctor's appointments and read extensively on all the literature about the operation. It would serve me well later.

I was very excited for the first time in years. I had followed the strict guidelines to a tee and now felt good about my selection to undergo the surgery. I realized this was not going to be a quick fix in getting thin but I had least been disciplined enough to follow all the preliminary steps required by the doctor. This became a continuing line of thought for I needed all the reinforcement I could muster. I felt the operation was a perfect fit for me. I had read and tried all approaches to "portion control." The use of smaller plates or waiting an hour after eating a meal to eat again had not worked for me. I had researched and attempted all these suggestions. And they had not worked for me. A surgery that would limit my ability to eat large amount of food seemed perfect for me.

On a side note, I had always eaten healthy foods. I ate very little red meat and usually bought organic and non-processed items to eat. There are many natural food stores in my home town of Westport and I was a frequent customer. I ate a lot of oatmeal and salads. I did occasionally binge on salty foods: popcorn, potato chips and those delicious cheddar cheese goldfish crackers. But overall I ate well. The problem was the amount I ate and the time of day I ate it. Sometimes I would stray. After spinning class, sometimes I would stop by the local bakery and choke down two delicious (and huge!) cinnamon rolls. My problem was definitely portion control and with menopause, my metabolism seemed to have virtually stopped.

Photo Gallery

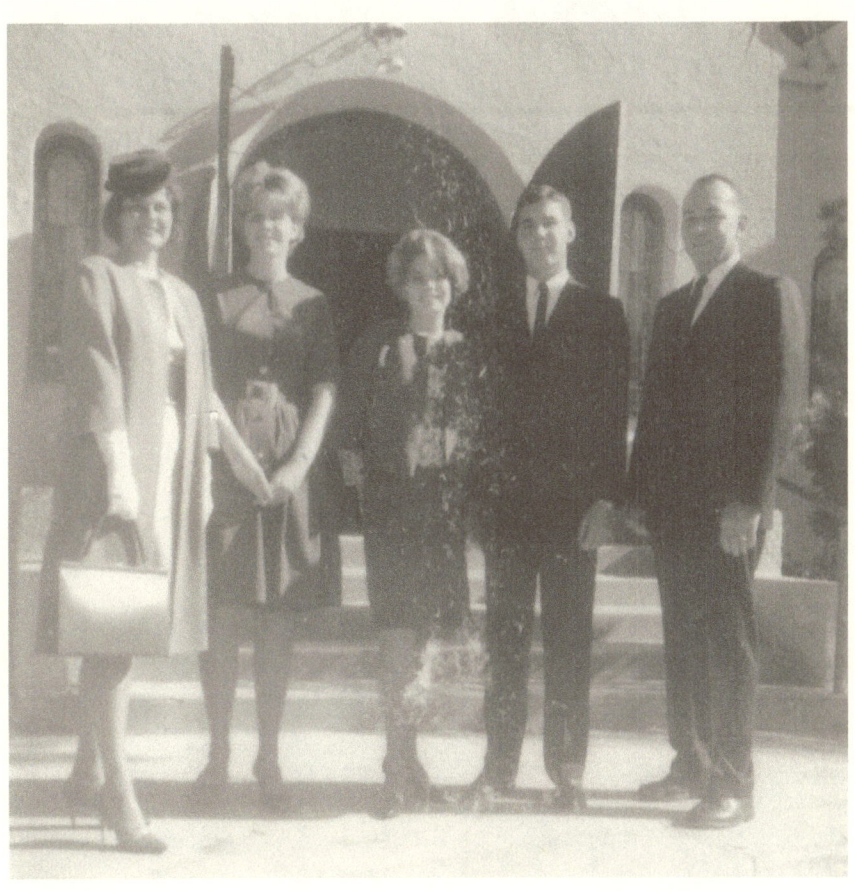

Our family at Christmas in California, 1963. I am in the middle and as you can see, I was the "shrimp" of the family. My father and mother are to the far right and left, respectively. I am flanked by my sister, Jacque and brother, Donald. Don was killed in a motorcycle accident only two months after this picture was taken.

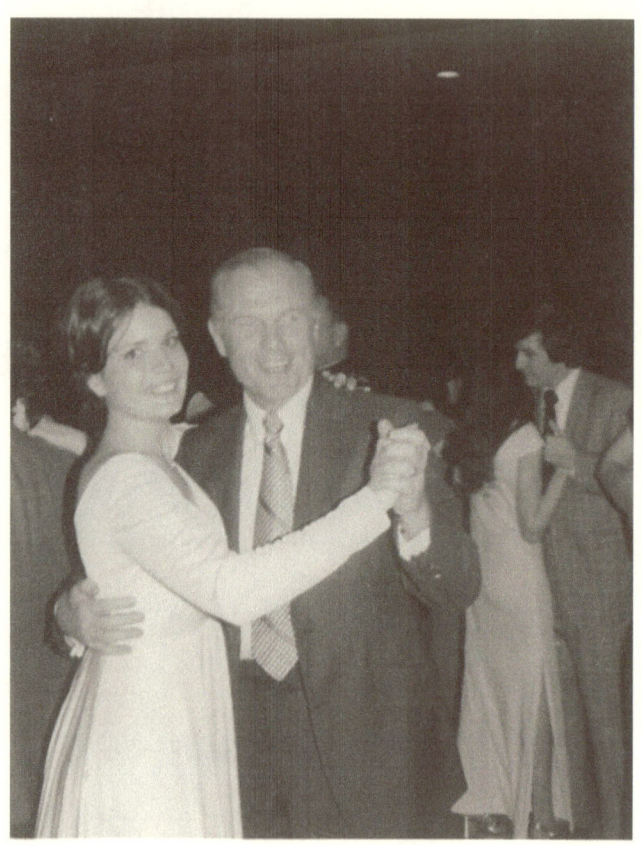

My wedding at Fort Monmouth in New Jersey, 1974, A very special dance with Uncle Johnny. People tried to "crash" the reception to get a good look at the first American to orbit the earth! What a great guy!

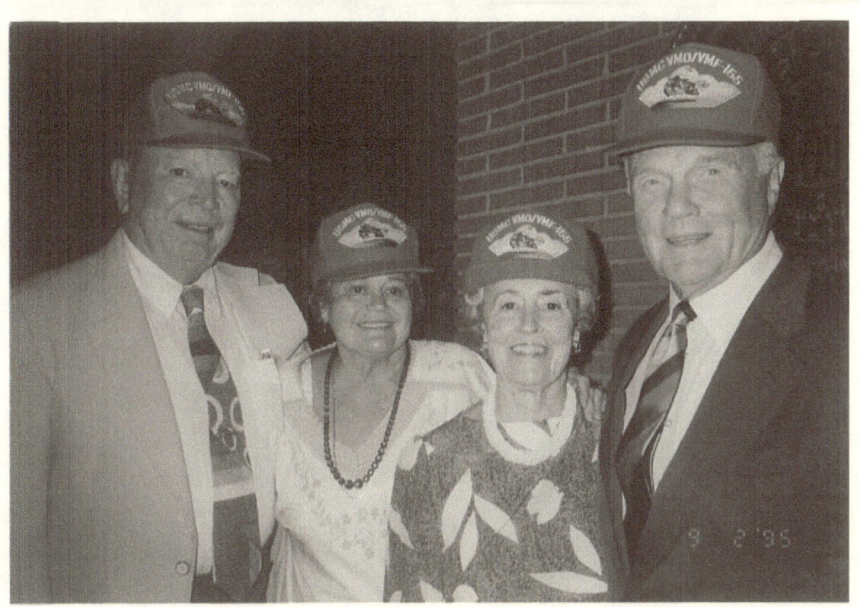

Mom and Dad with the Glenn's: "Aunt" Annie and "Uncle Johnny" in 1995. Dad and Senator Glenn went to flight school together in 1941 and flew in the same squadron in World War II and Korea. They were very much Marine brothers!

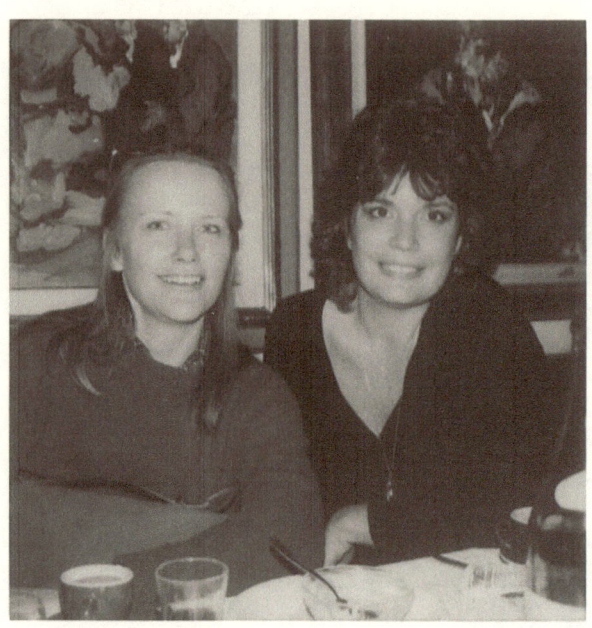

I traveled throughout most of Europe and Asia as an executive for the retail gi-
ant, Bamberger's. I loved the experience and the travel but it had its low points
too. Here I am with my assigned "interpreter in Florence, Italy, 1980.

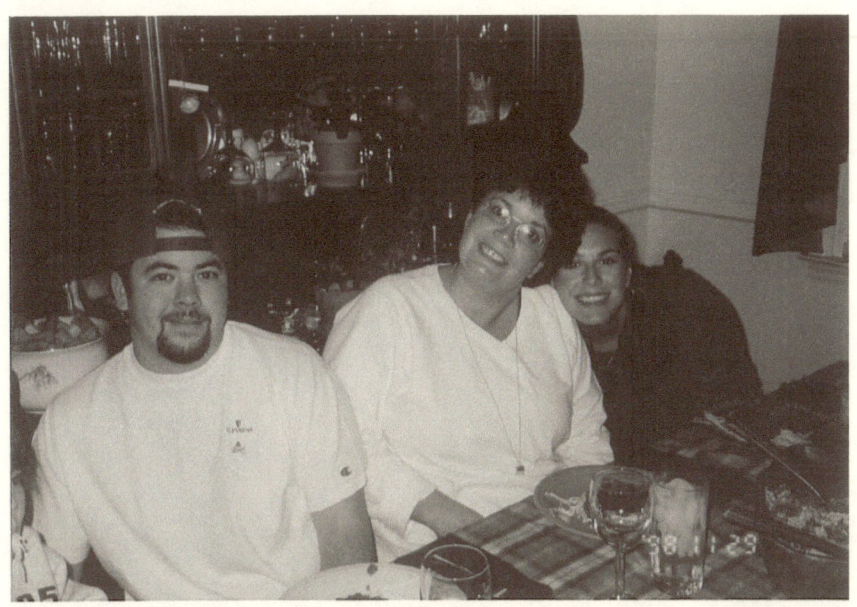

One of my favorite activities --- DINNER!! I was a realtor by now in Connecticut and living well. But the pounds were beginning to add up. I am with my godson, Ted Philpott and good friend, Krista O'Malley in this shot.

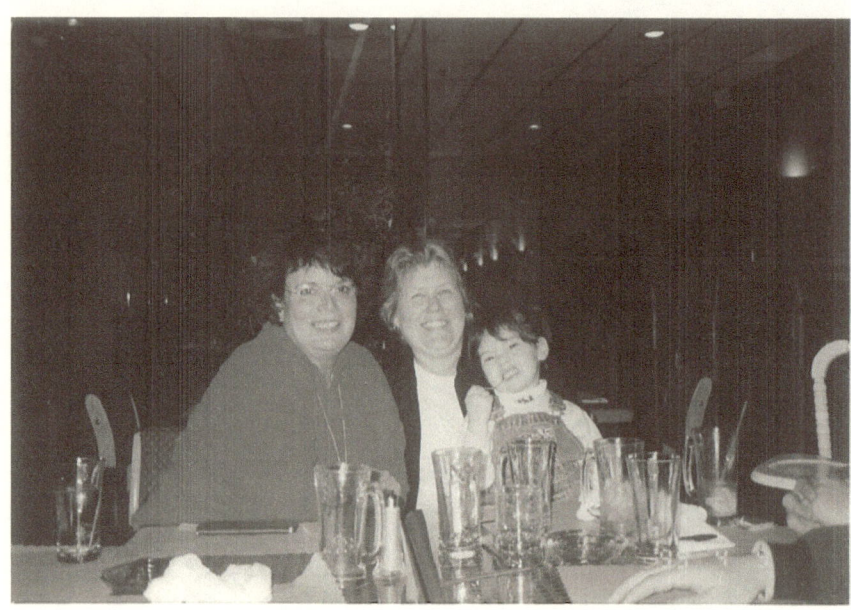

By 2001, I was at my heaviest, nearing 270 pounds! I am out to lunch in this picture with my best of best friends, Jane Philpott and her granddaughter, Kassidy.

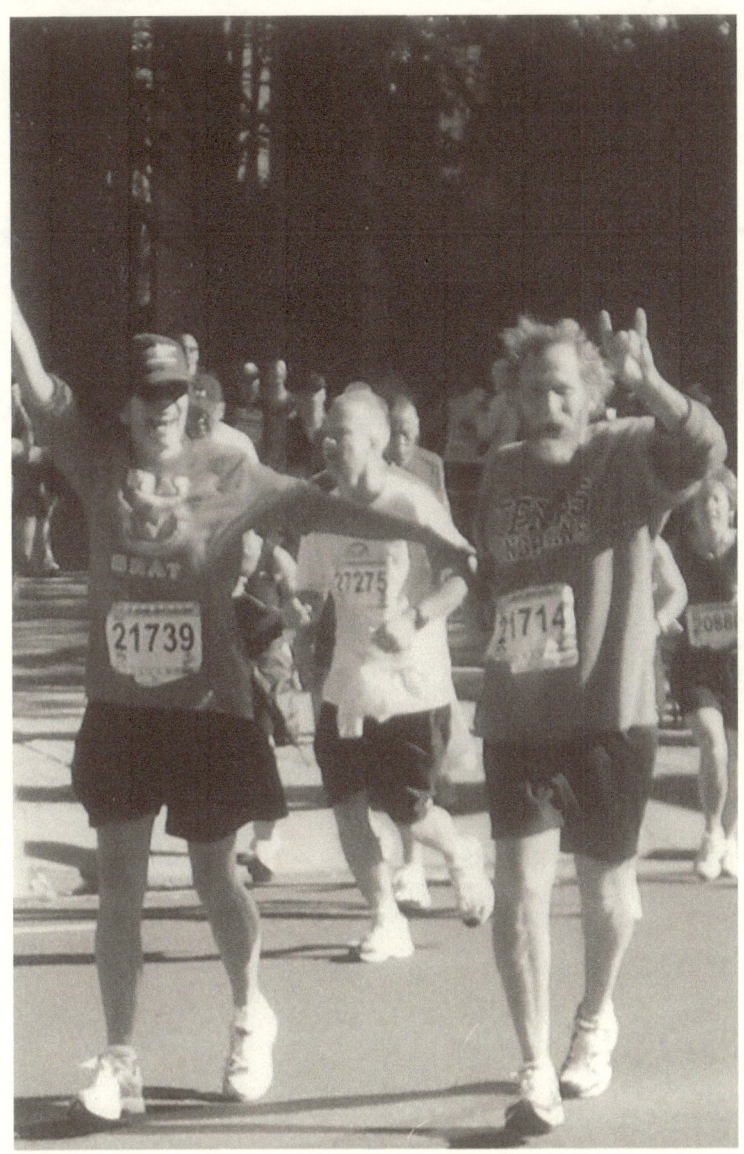

This picture was taken at mile 23 of the 2006 Marine Corps Marathon. I may not show it but I was tired and hurting. I found encouragement from the Philpott clan who came all the way from Connecticut to cheer me on!

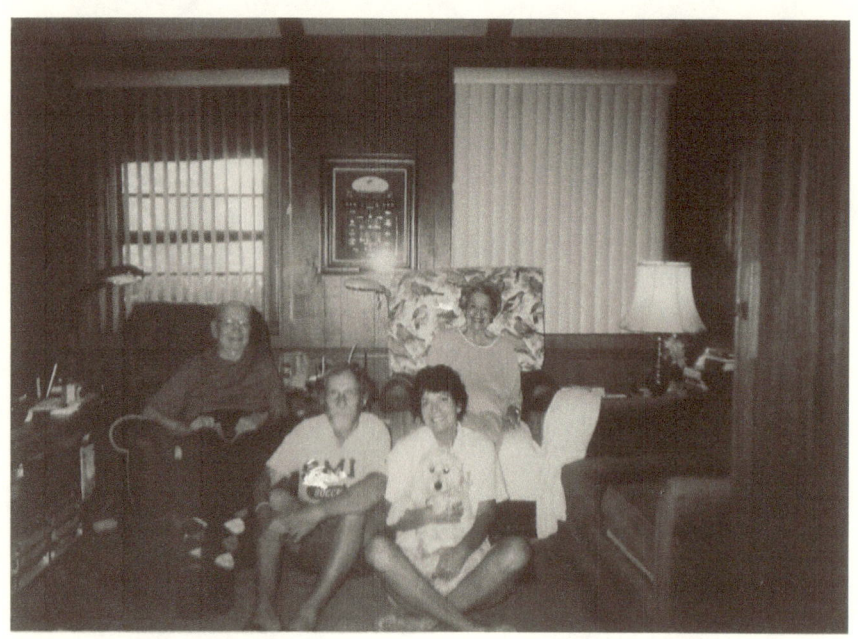

Mom and Dad, Carl and me at the Arlington home. We had a wonderful summer with them in 2006. Each would begin to fail in health after this time period. That is "TAZ", their wonderful little dog.

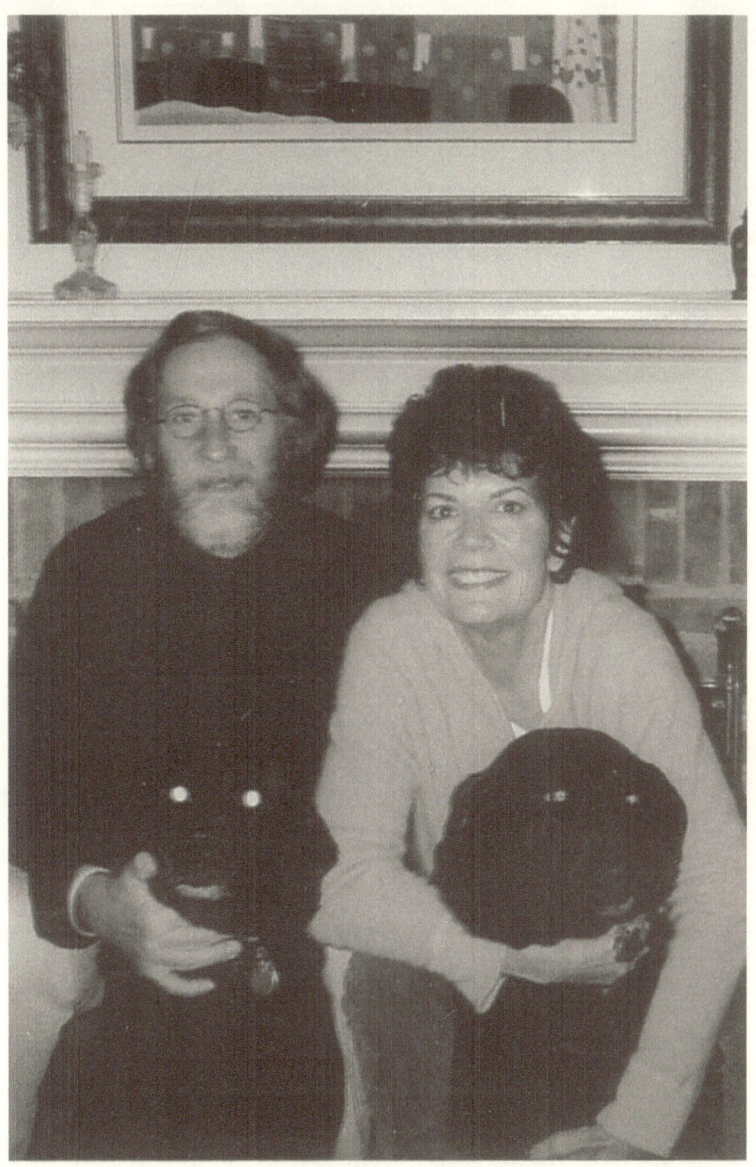

Carl and me with my dogs, Annie and Ben at Thanksgiving, 2006.

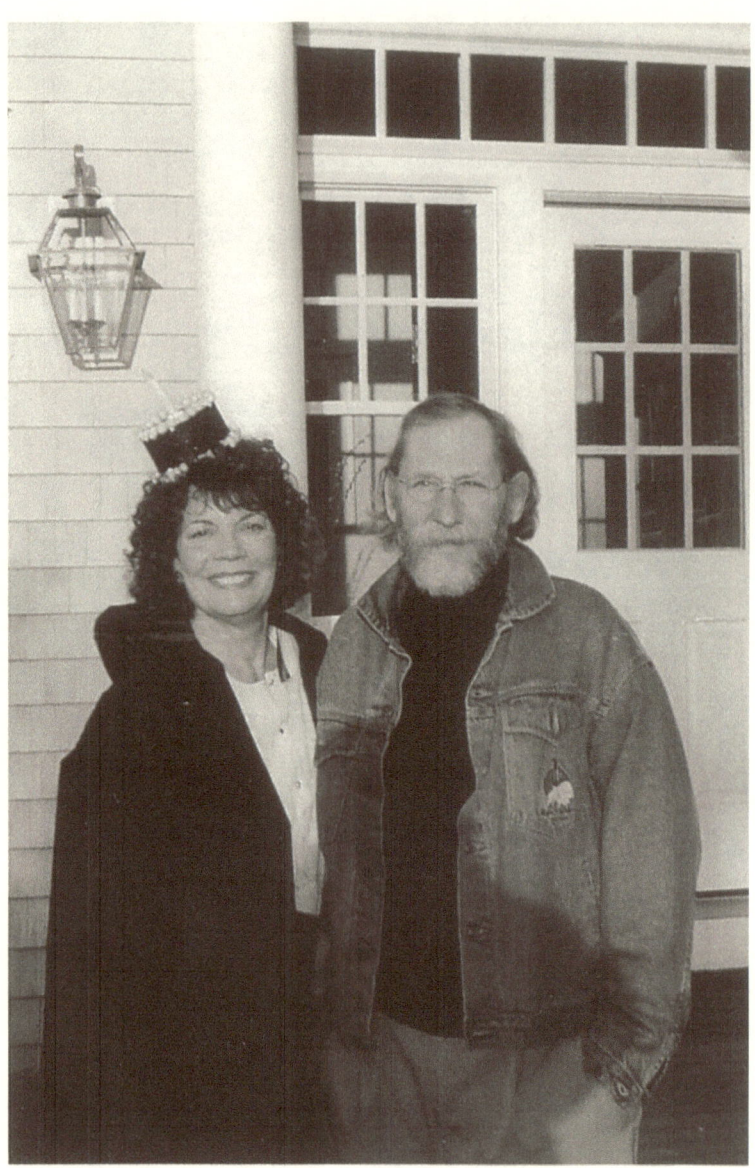

This is Carl and me on my 59th birthday at Cape Cod, Massachusetts. My good friend, Cindy Harper (and my best "reader") took this shot. Starting to think about the New York Marathon in 2010!

"Our thinking and our behavior are always in anticipation of a response. It is therefore fear-based."

Deepak Chopra

While the beautiful Lincoln Memorial lurked to my left, I began to feel bored with the race. The crowds were good and the surroundings spectacular, but I was getting tired of running. I was not necessarily physically tired but I was getting down on myself. In the first half of the race, I felt anticipation and excitement. The reality of the race had now set in and there was a very long way to go. I had been forewarned about this lull. The physical exhaustion was to come but the mental side was now taking its toll on my motivation. The race seemed endless.

Looking back, it was my positive approach to the idea of the surgery that really helped me make the decision to have the operation. I have always been an "up" person. I see the "glass of water half full." I have been called a "Pollyanna" too. While I feel I am also realistic and practical, I do confess to trying to see the best in people and the circumstances of life. Being obese was a downer but I was certainly not depressed or sad. I was very frustrated, however. Therefore, as I awaited the insurance company's and doctor's decision, I felt that my overall health, my love of exercise and physical activity, my choice of foods to eat and my overall positive attitude, were all major pluses to my selection.

I told everybody close to me except for my parents, sister and Joey. I did not want them to worry and maybe try to talk me out of it. I did tell one friend and he responded: "You are fine just the way you are." Well, I didn't want to be just "fine" and I knew I wasn't anyhow. After that, I was very selective about who I told. I wanted positive reinforcement and not any "naysayers." I didn't want any negative karma in my life.

I had done my homework and I was aware of the risk and possible complications. I was confident that the surgery was the right for me. Thus, for one of very first times in my life, I did not care what other people thought. This was very refreshing and allowed a sense of freedom to prevail over my thoughts. However, I still harbor some feelings of embarrassment that I had to resort to surgery to control my weight. But when I realized that I was really doing something very constructive in my life, my inhibitions went away. I recall telephoning my Aunt Lucy and telling her that I was going through some "minor surgery." She knows me very well and asked me if I was telling her the whole truth. I lied but ten minutes later I called her back and told her the whole story.

I finally received the good news when I was returning from my nephew's high school graduation near Boston. I got a call on my cell phone that I had been accepted! I had a surgery date. I cannot describe the feeling. The news made me feel like a little kid at Christmas. I turned on a CD and drove home for two hours listening to the loud music with a big smile on my face.

I had a final sit-down with my surgeon. The euphoria of being selected had been replaced with some reservations. I needed some reassurance that this was going to work. I also had read that nearly 20 percent of those undergoing this operation do not make it. They die! I found out later that this was not true. The percentage is actually less than one percent. The doctor spoke candidly with me. There were some risks to the surgical procedure but with my vital signs being in good shape, I was not at serious risk. And he reminded me of all the seminars that I had attended and the people I had met who had been successful losing weight following the surgery. He calmed my nerves.

My surgery was set for July 27, 2005. It had been a long three months in coming but in reflection, I am glad I took my time and made certain this was right for me. I was well on my way to my new beginning.

"Surgery is by the far worst snob among the handicrafts."

Austin O'Malley

We were leaving the down town mall area and heading out west of the city. The crowds were still good but my mood had not changed. I was normally fairly even keeled but today I was up and down emotionally. I knew I was taxing my body and that might affect my body chemistry. Through my months of training, I had become very familiar with the changes in your mind and body while you run the race. Thus I knew that my blood sugar was probably way low and made a mental note to take some oranges at the next water station. Part of being healthy or getting healthy is to learn. My running partner, who often refuses to go to the doctor, says he knows his body better than anyone else. I liked that philosophy and had attempted to learn as much as my mind would absorb.

Gastric Bypass Surgery is referred to as GBP by the doctors was developed in the 1960's by Doctor Edmund Mason to treat obese partners. According to April Hochstasser, Ph.D., in her **The Patient's Guide to Weight Loss Surgery - Revised:**

Gastric Bypass is a procedure in which a small gastric pouch is made in the small part of the upper stomach. The stomach is then severed at that point and forms scar tissue once healed. The larger portion of stomach is sealed off and the outlet to the small intestine remains. This leaves a small, blind pouch into which food arrives from esophagus.

Simply put, food that is eaten bypasses your big tummy and ends up in a little round pouch that is the size of your fist. You can't eat as much because of the small stomach as you lose weight.

In 2005, there were over 140,000 such operations completed in the United States. Over the years, various techniques have been developed to perform the operation. A very common technique and the type I had done is laparoscopy. To be exact, it is called the Laparoscopic Roux-en-Y Gastric Bypass (LRYGB) and it is considered to be the "gold standard" procedure by the American Society of Bariatric Surgeons. When the gastric bypass is done with this procedure, 5 to 7 small incisions are made. A camera, called a laparoscope, and long surgical instruments are used while the belly is inflated with carbon dioxide gas. The surgeon then operates while visualizing the internal organs on the television screen. During the LRYGB, a 30-60cc pouch is created by stapling-off the stomach. The remaining stomach stays alive and intact, and the far end is attached to the small bowel. This "remnant stomach" receives blood and produces digestive stomach acid. A 40 centimeter section of small bowel is then measured, cut, and reattached to the stomach by stapling, hand stitching, or a combination of the two. Another 100-200 centimeter of small bowel is then attached to the side of the limb to drain the new, small stomach portion.

There are several also other variations to the basic GBP: Roux en-Y (proximal), Roux en-Y (distal) and the Loop Gastric bypass. The most common is the "proximal" where the small bowel is divided below the lower stomach outlet and is rearranged into a Y-configuration. This allows for the greatest amount of nutrition to be derived from consumed food. In the "distal" method, the Y-connection is formed at the lower end of the bowel. This may deter the proper absorption of necessary nutriments through the stomach linings. Also used is the Loop Gastric bypass or mini-gastric bypass where a small loop of the small bowel for reconstruction rather than the Y-construction. Many bariatric surgeons have abandoned this method for there is distinct risk of leakage.

Gastric bypass surgery reduces the size of an average stomach by 90%. The stomach pouch erected is about the size of a man's fist. The surgery locates the pouch in an area where it is least susceptible to stretching. The pouch remains much the same over time but the size of the connection between the stomach and bowel may increase and allow the small bowel to hold more food. Usually, the loss of weight and acquired new eating habits preclude increased corruption of food. Thus, the fear of returned weight gain is diminished. It remains the responsibility of the patient, however, to learn and maintain new eating habits.

The above description is my own interpretation of what I have read and what I have been told. In no way should it be construed as medical advice or a definitive description of gastric bypass. You should consult your doctor on such issues.

MILE **16**

This was beginning to be no fun! We had left the good cheering crowds of the capitol area and now were moving to the outskirts of town. We headed down a roundabout loop in a state park to the east side of Washington. This was no man's land. Not a soul was there except for the occasional Marine or dear sweet volunteer. God Bless the volunteers!!! The pain in the upper side of my back, just beneath my neck was hurting. I wasn't sure where this was coming from and it worried me a bit. New pains meant new problems. And I didn't need any problems at the moment, thank you. It was warm but I was hydrated. The worse thing about this stretch was all my thoughts about my hurting body!

On my surgery day in July of 2005, it was hotter than hell. A good friend, Joe, drove me to the hospital and watched over me like a mother hen. He was comforting but I was not scared. My fears had been washed away by my reassuring doctor. I was actually somewhat excited about getting the operation over with and starting a new life. That may sound completely contrived but it was my state of mind.

I was convinced that this was a good thing for me and my Marine background didn't allow for any cowardice. I had gone through a disciplined regiment ten days prior to the surgery. I was only allowed 1,000 calories in food intake each day and six days after this period, I was only allowed clear liquids and broth. I am sure the temptation to splurge on a last eating binge would be great for many. But I was assured this regiment was absolutely necessary to the success of the surgery. Like the good "Marine" that I was, I followed orders to a tee.

I was alone in the pre-op room. Lying on the hospital bed, I thought of stories I had heard about patients changing their mind about the surgery just before the scheduled time. I imagined myself running out of the room with my butt hanging out of the gown!

Doctor Floch arrived shortly thereafter. Once again he was re-assuring. Soon needles went into my arm and I was getting woozy. I woke up four hours later in the recovery room feeling sort of dopey but extremely happy. I was smiling and glad to have the surgery over. Doctor Floch was there by my side telling me that everything had gone according to plan and asking me how I felt. "Perfect," I replied.

The first part of the journey had come to an end. I had stuck with the required preoperative program and done well. Thanks to a good doctor and staff of the Fairfield County Bariatrics, I had remained focused. I had accomplished what I had set out to do. This was important. My positive mindset continued to help me.

I have learned that there is a very definite psychological effect to preparing for and undergoing LYYGB surgery. Many people suffering from obesity lose any sense of accomplishment. They, and I include myself, feel powerless to the food that makes us sick. As a result, we fall prey to becoming depressed and afraid of change. The fear comes from our failure to stop the weight gain and that emotion often snowballs to affect all parts of one's life.

My upbringing, however, did not allow me to wallow in self-pity so my low moods were limited. But many are not as fortunate as I had been. While, the completion of the surgery made me feel good about myself, now it was the time to make it work!

MILE **17**

"Surgery is half the race but you have to do the follow-up or you do yourself a major disservice."

Fran Drescher

The route down the peninsula through the government property continued. It seemed endless. I began to walk for the first time. I felt exhausted. I knew I had to keep going for there was no place to turn back. When there is a turnaround, you can see the runners ahead of you and this is not good. For one they look terrible by this stage of the race and second, you realize that they are at least one mile or so ahead of you. Also, I didn't know where the turnaround was for I did not know the course very well. Many elite athletes drive the course prior to running it. That gives you a good idea of how far the loop really is or how big the hill might be. I didn't do this because I certainly knew I was not going to get lost by being the first runner. In retrospect I should have become more familiar with the race course. But all this marathon stuff was new to me

After the surgery, my great doctor allowed me to go home a day early. I had been there only two days. I was not good in hospitals. I was antsy and to be confined to a bed all the time was not my idea of fun. So, thank you Doctor Floch for understanding my mind as well as my body. It was great to hear those choice few words: "You can go home today."

My good friend and co-worker, Carol, picked me up at the hospital. She was the best. Not only did she wait on me hand and foot but she had a "special gift" for me. She and some other close friends had gone to Victoria Secret and bought me some very skimpy underwear! The panties were so small in size, that they would have fit a skinny teenager! I laughed so hard I started to cry. It was the perfect gift for someone who had just gone through gastric bypass surgery. Now all I had to do was fit into them!

If you think the work is done when you have the surgery, think again. As I have indicated, the diet preceding the operation was fairly strict: 1,000 calories a day ten days prior to my surgery and six days into that, I only could have clear liquids like broth or soup. Now I was told I had to repeat that regiment plus insure that I had 82 grams of protein in my diet every day. Oh, my dear!

I wasn't really that hungry but food looked very good. It smelled even better. In my mind I thought I could have definitely eaten a big steak and a baked potato. But I stuck to my guns and followed the doctor's orders. I was being good and figured that I had invested this much time and money in getting thin, I would listen to my doctor.

The post operative stage is a downfall for many people. They tend to think that they can eat anything when they immediately come from the operating table. But the doctors want you to slowly readjust to your new stomach. They also want you to lose fat but not muscle mass. So once again, I was slowly eating broth and sipping on clear protein drinks and water.

There are some specific complications that can arise following GBP. There can be some leakage from the gastrointestinal tract into the abdominal cavity. This can lead to infection. There also can be some constriction in the flow of food when scar tissue

forms in the new stomach. The diet of clear liquids can help healing and avoid these two problems. Doctors are also concerned
about nutritional deficiencies. Since patients are eating less, they
are taking in reduced calories and therefore, less good nutrition.
There are deep concerns regarding nutritional deficiencies following the surgery. Calcium supplements are needed for fear of
weakened and broken bones. Protein intake is needed to avoid
muscle loss, serious illness and skin problems. Iron deficiency is
also a concern. Problems may lead to dizziness, chronic fatigue
and low blood count. Daily iron supplements are needed to avoid
such issues. B-12 and B-1 are also needed to eliminate the possibility of paralysis and nerve damage. Vitamin and mineral levels
in your blood must be monitored at least twice yearly by your
physician. Unfortunately, most of these supplements come in pill
form. I found that I had to crush the pills or take liquid vitamins in
order to not only get them down but to digest them. Once again,
I remind you that this is what I have learned and worked for me. It
should not be considered as medical advice.

I never weighed myself before returning to the doctor after two
weeks. I was afraid that I would be disappointed in my progress if
I weighed myself. So when I jumped on the scale at the doctor's
office and learned that I had lost 30 pounds, I was elated! I also
received permission to start eating solid foods.

Immediately, I went to the store to buy some food. My refrig-
erator had been empty for too long. For some unknown reason,
I bought a bunch of humus. That was my first meal. It tasted like
a filet mignon. I loved it. I didn't much like humus before and not
much now. But that meal was memorable. At the time, I honestly
thought the surgery had changed my taste buds along with the
size of my stomach.

For the first few weeks I had no problems with the digestion
of food. I ate very slowly and cautiously. When I ate too fast, the
food would get stuck and I would have to stop. It was a little scary
at first but I eventually got use to food taking longer to get down

into my stomach. I tried to eat slower and really chew my food well. I watched what kind of food I ate. I tried to stay away from processed foods and I continued to eat soft foods. If I ate too close to bed time, I would have to sleep sitting up for fear that the food would regurgitate. I also had a problem with liquids. If I gulped my usual bottle of water, it would not go down. One time I was driving and took a huge swallow of water. I had to stop the car and get out, and threw up the water. It just would not go down. I had to relearn how to eat, when to eat and what to put in my mouth. It was the exact purpose of the surgery. To make you THINK!!!!

One problem suffered by many GBP patients is called "dumping." It occurs when you eat a sugar-filled food and the sugar passes quickly into the bowel. The sugar sends a message to your mind that triggers all sorts of terrible things. Your heart begins to race, you break into a cold sweat and you really think that you are going to throw up. About six months after my surgery, my personal trainer, Julie, brought an Angel food cake when she visited for dinner. As I remember, we had a simple dinner of fish and rice. I didn't have room for desert that night but the next night, I indulged in just a sliver of the cake. Wow! I had to run for the bedroom to sit down. It felt like I was having a heart attack. But I calmed myself down and began to focus on breathing very slowly. After about 30 minutes, I was fine. It did teach me a permanent lesson: no more sweets. I found a no-sugar blueberry pie at the local supermarket and have found it a great substitute.

If you do not eat properly for a long period of time, there is the possibility of reversing the effects of the operation. If a GBP patient returns to his or her prior eating habits or to overeating, there is a good chance that the stomach will begin to stretch and allow for more and more food to be digested. As a result, whatever weight that was lost may return. This has to be disheartening but this information is known to everyone undergoing the operation prior to the surgery. GBP is not a magic pill. It is a means to an end. One has to relearn new disciplines in their life to be successful in permanent weight loss. This is difficult for many of us who were not really good about being disciplined before the surgery. But it is absolutely necessary to be successful.

MILE **18**

"When we are tired, we are attacked by ideas we conquered long ego."

Friedrich Nietzche

The lackluster loop continued and I was walking and running now. I was just suddenly tired. My whole body ached and I wondered if this was the "wall" that everyone had told me about. At this juncture, your glycogen or sugar level hits bottom and you just do not have enough energy. I took a finger full of the honey in my little bagey in my pocket. My mood was suddenly better but I was still tired.

I was now on the return section of the loop and could see runners where I had been some twenty minutes earlier. For some reason that made me feel better. I was ahead of a lot of people. The competitive side of me got me running again although the scenery still remained boring.

I had been running for nearly three hours now and it had taken its toll on my mind. My body had some pains here and there but I knew I had to overcome the mental depression. I took some more honey and it hit the spot. I gained some strength and felt motivated. My mind returned to my post-surgery transformation.

As the months went by and the pounds began to disappear, I got into a daily routine as to eating. I found that fluffy doughy foods did not sit well. I had never liked greasy fatty foods so that was not a problem. In the morning, I started the day with a protein shake with many vitamins and supplements. After I learned that there were issues with nutrition and the post-surgery, I contacted a naturopathic doctor. For those unfamiliar, naturopathy is a method of treating disease, using food, exercise and vitamins to assist the natural healing process. I was told to continue with my surgeon's recommendations of calcium, B-12, B-1 and iron but also to add a multiple vitamin each day with fish oil capsules, and a healing agent, acidophilius. I also took several herbs including bioflavonoid maxifulux and mushroom nutritional tablets. These helped balance my nutritional needs and helped the absorption of deficient vitamins to my body. Supplements may vary per individual patient, so consult your doctor.

I ate salad every day for lunch. I chopped up kale, spinach, baby lettuce and/or romaine lettuce in small pieces by using scissors along with cutup mushrooms and cheese. It is excellent to the taste and for your fiber intake. Dinner was usually salmon, steak, sometimes quiche (egg whites only) or occasionally, Mexican tacos. I had "no sugar added" blueberry pie with whipped cream for dessert sometimes or sugar free popsicles. I never ate very late at night.

The doctors tell you NOT to "graze" with food but I ate constantly in the morning or when I traveled. I snacked on peanut butter and natural cheese. In addition, whenever I traveled I took my own food. I did not want to tempt myself with junk food or fast food chains. I premade salads and took a large container of natural peanut butter with me. I also ate deboned and range free skinless chicken.

As mentioned, all the doctors tell you to watch your protein intake. I was advised to eat at least 82 grams of protein a day.

This amount was based on my weight. I began to replace my protein shake with oatmeal and cottage cheese for breakfast. I ate cheese a lot. Within four months, I had increased my intake of beef, chicken and fish. My drink of choice was water. I was never a juice fan or soda junkie so it was not hard to stick with the no calorie water. I did drink decaffeinated coffee in the morning. I love coffee. I also drank a glass of wine with dinner but found that more than a glass gave me the shakes the next day so I watch how much I drink.

Immediately after the surgery, I had trouble sleeping. While I was heavy, I was tested for sleep apnea and was found I suffered from it. This is where you actually stop breathing during sleep. During my test, I stopped breathing 52 times in a six hour period. This was related to my obesity but is also a factor when you undergo any type of surgery. After my operation, I slept better but still was not getting complete sleep. My primary doctor prescribed me 1 mg of Xanax to take at bedtime. So I take one of these pills and several chewable calcium tablets at night and I sleep super! I should caution everyone that Xanax can become habit forming but I have been taking it for three years now and I never need more than that one pill.

By mid-October, some three months after my surgery, I had lost over 75 pounds. I felt extremely good and everybody told me I looked wonderful. My goal was another fifty pounds but then . . .

"Everybody wants to get old but nobody wants to be old."

John Wolfgang Van Goethe

There is the infamous story of how the marathon began and for some reason it popped into my mind. The folklore goes that a guy named Pheidippides, back in 490 B.C., ran exactly 26.2 miles to report the outcome of the battle of Marathon. Upon announcing the victory of the Greeks, the messenger dropped dead. So this is supposedly why the marathon is 26.2 miles vice an even twenty-six. It is the distance from Marathon to Athens. The distance really doesn't matter to most folks but the fact that he dropped dead is an eye catcher. As I kept pounding away, walking some and then running, I could empathize with poor Pheidippides.

"Joey" had been my next door neighbor for over twenty years. He was a kind sweet man. He was in his early eighties but seemed older. He was a tall big man with a gentle face. His nose and ears were too big for his face but his eyes were sincere and caring. His smile would light up any room. Joey had been handsome when he was young but now had that calm, content grandfather look.

He grew up in my new hometown of Westport and had lived here his entire life. He joined the Army when he turned eighteen, just after the outbreak of World War II. Much like my father, he enlisted as soon as he could to come to the aid of America. He was a hero, fighting gallantly in New Guinea and on the Pacific front. After the war, he returned to Connecticut to become a postman.

Joey was a very caring individual and while very much the quiet loner, he was known by everyone in the tiny suburb. Joey never married. He lived with his sister, Helen, and her husband. They lived right next door to me and we actually shared a drive-way. He watched the town develop into an affluent suburb of New York City. I am not sure he liked all the change but he saw his house appreciate forty times its initial value. But Joey didn't much care about money. He was content in his small world of the Yankees, Rangers and looking out for me along with my two dogs.

When Joey's brother-in-law died of a heart attack and his sister Helen fell ill to Alzheimer's disease, Joey was very much alone. I went from being a close neighbor to being his family and his caretaker. Our two houses became one home. I would see him early every morning and every night after work. I made sure he was eating properly and helped him with anything he might need. Joey could still drive but he was forgetful. I made sure he was safe and had everything he needed. He was never demanding and was always so appreciative for everything I was doing. Joey was also not in the best of health. He suffered from heart disease stemming from having rheumatic fever as a child. He also had extremely bad knees which limited his mobility.

I did not tell Joey about my surgery for fear of him worrying too much. I told him that it was just a "female thing." We spent a lot of time together during my brief recovery period. I would bring him breakfast every morning from a nearby deli. He loved eggs and bacon on a Portuguese roll. We would sit at his kitchen table and talk about the Yankees. Joey's mind was not the best and he often repeated the same stories to me. But that was okay. I loved the man like a father. He watched over my two dogs while I was at work and I helped in any way I could. He was a very dear friend and he was really a surrogate father to me. I know he also loved me like a daughter he never had. We were a family.

After a week or two of my so-called rehabilitation, which was really taking it easy around the house, I was able to return to work. I felt fantastic and the pounds were slipping away. Not long after that, I took Joey for his annual physical with his local doctor. The news was not good. Joey's heart was only operating at a 35% rate of capacity. With his sly sense of humor, Joey asked: "Is that not good?" We laughed that day. It would be one of the last times we laughed together.

The doctor feared that Joey might suffer a heart attack at any time. He restricted his activity. Joey used a cane mostly because of his bad knees and drove to the store some but he really did not move around much. His day was usually spent sitting in a big arm chair staring out the front window. I always wondered what was going through his mind. He never talked much. He always loved to hear about me and my day. Joey loved my two new black Labrador retrievers "Ben" and "Annie." They spent each day with him. Joey also liked to feed the squirrels in the yard. He would give them peanuts every day as they flocked around his back door.

I think the doctor's words bothered me more than Joey. He just smiled and took the news with good spirit. That was Joey. I was worried. I had gone through hell with Joey's sister. Helen was very impatient with her mental deterioration and became very angry. She wandered off and we found her once two miles away. She just kept walking. I had to basically quit work and take care of her. For a time, I actually had to live off my credit cards and borrow money from my father to get by. I didn't really think I had a choice. My neighbors were my extended family. But now it was somewhat different. Joey was alone and I was coming off major surgery plus my parents were now suffering from health problems. Work was still demanding and I needed some form of income to make ends meet. I was in the middle of a hard balancing act when all of a sudden an angel appeared . . .

"Coincidences are God's way of remaining anonymous."

Albert Einstein

George Shehan, the original guru of running, once wrote that "anyone can run twenty miles but not everyone can run a marathon." I was at that point now with my run. The next six miles would be on "sheer guts" according to the guru. My body was diminishing in strength. I was tired after nearly four hours of constant running, I was hungry and hot. Other than that, everything was fine.

We hit the cut off mark at the 14th Street Bridge with plenty of time to spare. There was a four hour and 30 minute cutoff time. I hated to think of some of those held behind of the delayed start that would be picked up by Marines with their races finished. To run twenty miles and be turned away didn't seem fair but those were the rules.

The crowds were crazy underneath the bridge and I ran through a narrow line of spectators that felt like I was competing at the Tour de France. It was crazy fun and I got my mind off my sour mood and tired body. Six miles to go. Running beside me the whole way was the love of my life.

In the fall of 1967 when I was lowly "fresh person" in college, I had a date with a sophomore soccer player who was athletic, had wild blond hair and was very cute. We only went out once. He took me to a fraternity party and I got pretty drunk on two beers. We ended up "making out" in the chapel until the wee hours of the night, well past curfew. College girls had curfews in those "olden" days. The next morning I felt somewhat embarrassed about the extent of the after-date session, so I told him that I had a crush on one of his fellow soccer players and just wanted to be friends. This was partially true but I think I was more concerned about my reputation than anything else. In those days, the "loose" label was something you wanted to avoid. He was pretty wild back then too. He would soon get booted from college for nearly running over an assistant Dean after driving through the school's dormitory quadrangle area. Needless to say, he had been drinking. So we never dated again and soon he was drafted into the military and serving in Vietnam.

Some thirty-eight years later, this same cute soccer player called me just after the news about Joey's heart and also, my surgery. "Carl" was living in Vermont, teaching golf. He had just returned from a mini-college reunion where he found an alumni book that listed my name and address. What caught his interest was that I now lived in his hometown of Westport. He found this "too hard to believe" and decided he must call me. He sounded very interesting but to tell you the truth, I didn't remember him very well at all. I gave him my email address and didn't think much about it.

The next morning I received an email from him. He revealed that he was recovering from the break-up of a long term marriage and living in his grandfather's house in northern Vermont. He had lived in Texas for many years and practiced law there. He was now a writer, sometimes golf pro and living a very simple and seemingly lonely lifestyle. His emails, which would continue, were funny and laced with a flirtation that made me feel special. I endured many emotions during my obesity and leading up to the surgery but my intimate sexuality were not among them. They had been stored in reserve for quite some time. I am not sure if being overweight was a way I kept from having to deal with this type of emotion. Whatever the reasons, I was enjoying the playfulness of our electronic relationship. I checked my computer often to see if I had received an email from him.

My parents were always very strong in their faith and Christian tradition. I had attended church much of my life. I taught Sunday school. Yet, I never considered myself a devout follower of the church. I believed in a good force and spirit. I just wasn't sure where it came from. However, the day Carl called and really came into my life, I received a firm contract on a house that I was selling. It turned out to be the exact property that his parents had owned while he was growing up. This was so coincidental it was almost eerie. It was as if some divine power was sending an angel to me.

Carl was aggressive. The words "we can be friends" that I said to him 38 years ago was not what he wanted to hear now. It seemed strange to me that he seemed to know that he wanted to pursue a relationship with me without having seen each other for so long. He wanted to meet and not just communicate via email. I was still losing weight and was not comfortable enough with my own self image to arrange a date. I put him off. The email electronic relationship began to flourish.

His emails became the highlight of my day. I have never been much of a writer but I was enjoying the communication. We certainly got to know each other rather quickly and probably faster than we would have in person. I also was not only learning a lot about Carl but about myself. I had never experienced having to write down my inner most feelings. He was very inquisitive about my personal self and curious about my life. I found myself writing long emails about things I have rarely shared with anyone before. It was very therapeutic at a time in my life when I certainly needed it. He made me feel very special.

Carl called after a month of emailing. Hearing his voice put a new perspective on our relationship. He became a real person with a real voice and not just mail on my computer. It was strange going from reading his words to now listening to a voice. It added another dimension to our relationship. It was definitely more personal. He was funny and I liked that. We teased each other and flirted like teenagers. It was silly but fun and exciting at the same time. The only problem he was moving a bit fast for me. I was still dealing with the physical changes and self image issues resulting from my surgery. There was a sense of trepidation and insecure feelings attached to my size. I didn't feel very comfortable with my body. When I underwent the surgery and began to lose weight, I gained a sense of real hope. I was looking forward to not being so self-conscious of my looks. I just wanted to feel good about the way I looked. The relationship with Carl brought this instinct alive. I had not been with a man for five years and while I thought I did not need the intimacy of a relationship, I found myself very much interested. I may have used my weight as an excuse not to pursue relationships. That was behind me now.

I had never thought I needed a man in my life, but I was beginning to enjoy the companionship that we were sharing emailing and the phone calls. Maybe I did want a man in my life? I had not really thought about this in over twenty years. That may sound trite or old fashioned especially coming from a career woman. But it was true. Carl seemed like a go-to guy. When he mentioned that he would be working on a novel with his agent in New York City in the coming months, I suggested that he stay with Joey. I knew that Joey could use the company and the supervision. It would also give me a chance to really get to know Carl.

We met on Columbus Day, three months after my surgery. I had lost about seventy pounds by then but I was still pretty "robust". Carl surprised me when he made an unexpected trip in from the city. I rushed home when he called from Joey's and quickly changed into a deep purple cashmere sweater that I thought looked flattering. Carl was cute with a scruffy beard and a Robin Williams look about him. His glasses didn't hide his deep blue eyes. I was not overwhelmed but I was smitten. I gave him a big kiss when we said goodbye. Later he would say that the kiss sealed the deal. Our emails and phone conversations had rekindled a hidden sexuality within me. The relationship was fun, sexy and made me feel young and attractive. Carl kept me making me feel better and better about life. Life was good!

"Love is like energy. It can never be created or destroyed."

Ian Philpot

After the huge crowds at the entrance to the bridge, there was no one around on the bridge itself. I did some walking here. I was hurting and there was no question about this being me hitting the "wall." Physically spent. Emotionally drained. Hello marathon!

I was confident that I was going to finish. It was more of a feeling of when that would happen? I wanted this marathon to be over. This feeling of desperation apparently is not uncommon to runners at this stage of the race. There were many around me on the bridge that looked as tired as I did. I wanted to finish well, however. I had pride and didn't just want to walk the dang race. So when I got a yell of encouragement from one of the sweet Marines on the bridge, I started to run again with Carl right by my side.

Carl moved down from Vermont on the weekend before Halloween. We remained somewhat distant. We would later learn that we both were very shy! I had also emailed him that it was my custom to kiss everyone when they departed my home. How could I be so stupid? I felt like an idiot. Carl was smart as a whip. He had been a lawyer and now was a writer. Although he was never condescending to me, I felt inferior to him intellectually. As we got to know each other and communicated our beliefs and experiences, I realized that I was no dummy either. I think that is the most important part of a new relationship. That there is a side of you that perhaps you never knew existed. Carl was amazed at my knowledge of sports and how I put real estate deals together. It really gave me a new perspective of myself. I was gaining confidence and losing weight. I was down nearly 100 pounds by the time Halloween arrived.

The day after Halloween, Joey came down with a bad cough. After it persisted, I called Joey's primary doctor. He suggested an over-the-counter cough syrup. But when I tried to give it to Joey, he nearly went into convulsions. He could not swallow and I thought he was going into a seizure. Joey eventually caught his breath and seemed fine. Three days later, however, he was not eating and looked terrible. I decided to take him to the hospital. Carl came with us and his presence really was calming for me. I was so used to doing this type of thing alone. I had done it with my father, mother and Joey's sister. To have someone to share the stress of this situation was very comforting. It was another plus on the relationship side. I never thought I needed anyone in my life but now I knew I certainly enjoyed it. Carl really became my special angel during this period and I will forever be indebted to him.

Joey was diagnosed with having two strokes. I have no idea how they determined he had two but that was the explanation. Poor Joey couldn't swallow anything. He gagged on water. He was severely dehydrated and they admitted him to the hospital. I feared the worst. First, the news about his heart and now he had suffered strokes. I felt terribly anxious and while Carl was reassuring and good company, I needed time alone.

MILE **22**

"The life of inner peace, being harmonious and without stress, is the easiest type of existence."

Norman Vincent Peale

The marathon route took us in the back of the pack through Crystal City, a shopping area east of Arlington. It was full of people and the inward "ham" in me came out once again. I liked the support as if we all were a "team" taking me to the finish line. For once in my life, I was the center of a lot of attention and I was enjoying it.

My good friends, the Philpotts, had driven down from Connecticut especially for the race and I was anxious to see them. As always the "people pleaser", I was concerned about whether they were enjoying the marathon. I knew I didn't look at my best but they were such good friends, it really didn't matter. They were there, some fifteen strong and all dressed in yellow. We gave them all hugs and with their constant urging, we are were off again running. I always joke that I knew Jane Philpott before she was born because our parents were best of Marine friends. Both fathers were pilots and mothers good buddies. Jane and I continued that tradition, living very close to each other and best friends. She had recently gone through a divorce after thirty years of marriage. She had been hurt. I suddenly remembered my coping skills during the last year.

I had started a daily routine of meditation before my gastric bypass surgery. I carried a list of "symptoms of inner peace" with me which I plastered all over my home. When I was stressed out, I would sit down and read them. They are:

1. A tendency to thin and act spontaneously rather than fears based on past experiences;
2. An unmistakable ability to enjoy each moment;
3. A loss of interest in judging other people;
4. A loss of interest in conflict;
5. A loss of the ability to WORRY;
6. Frequent episodes of appreciation;
7. Feelings of contentment with others and nature;
8. Frequent attacks of smiling;
9. A tendency to let things happen rather than make them happen;
10. An increasing susceptibility to the love extended by others and an uncontrollable urge to extend it.

I found these ten descriptive symptoms in a book. I typed them up and put them in conspicuous places to insure I would read them often. While Joey lay in the hospital, I sat at the computer thinking of him and wanting to cry. Instead, I read my inner peace list. I have never been able to truly meditate or perform yoga. I have trouble sitting still let alone mastering my mindset. But reading this list helped me. I felt safe. I felt confident that Joey would be okay. The list was highly motivating and it helped me tremendously.

"Make friends with pain and you will never be alone."

Ken Chloubler

The slight euphoria of seeing my friends and the floodgate of support from the huge crowds around the mall was short-lived. For
by the 23rd mile marker, there was no one around. The Pentagon
was on my left and for security reasons, no access was available
for spectators. This was probably a good idea in my case for I was
getting in a lousy mood. I had begun to walk again, my left knee
hurting, my neck ached and my feet were sore. I had taken some
jelly beans from a Marine but it had little effect. My honey was
gone and I popped my last two Advils for the pain. I did not feel
like running at all. My juices had been spent. I was done. But then
I thought about Joey.

Joey came home for Thanksgiving. He had been on an in-
travenous feeding tube while he was at the hospital and gained
some weight back. He seemed to eat when he wanted to and had
little trouble swallowing but at most times, he wouldn't go near
food. I loved the holiday. It was my favorite and I loved to cook up

a storm and put out a feast. Carl had gone to New York City for the long weekend to work. I missed him but he was not the type of individual to keep restricted. He was going through a difficult period missing his own children and his career as a writer was in limbo. So I made do with my surrogate family. Joey sat at the head of the table. He ate well and I was so happy. He seemed so very content and comfortable being home. But it was not to last.

Joey took a turn for the worse after Thanksgiving. He slept most of the day and despite Carl's urgings, he did not eat much at all. It was not like Joey to share his thoughts. He was never a complainer. When his sister had died, he behaved much the same. But now, he withdrew from any communication and slept much of the day. Both Carl and I tried to get him out and about but Joey was having nothing to do with it. In retrospect, Joey may have made the decision to die. I am not sure people can really do this but I am sure that Joey had lost the will to live. I also think he believed Carl had arrived to take care of me and he could now let go. I know Joey felt a great responsibility toward me and did not want me to be by myself. I think Joey prayed for someone to come into my life. He did not want me to be by myself. Carl was the answer to his wishes. For a career woman, I know this sounds sexist but Joey was truly a chauvinistic type of guy. He was one of the good guys, my special guy.

Joey lost about fifteen pounds in a matter of weeks. He was painfully thin and the doctors wanted him back in the hospital. They hooked him up with an IV again and he did better. His physician recommended a feeding tube. This is an apparatus inserted surgically in one's stomach that allows for someone to be fed by pouring liquids through the tube directly into your stomach. It sounds simple but I think the doctors downplayed the seriousness and success of such a procedure. Joey had named me attorney-in-fact regarding any medical decisions. While Joey was coherent and could carry on intelligent conversations, his competency as to these decisions was questionable. He was a dear sweet man but his mind wandered and his intelligence had diminished with age. So with the help of attorney Carl and many conversations with Joey, I gave permission for the insertion of the feeding tube. The irony of the situation did not hit me until later. I just had an operation to stop me from eating too much and now Joey was undergoing a procedure that would allow him to eat more.

The operation was successful and after a few more days in the hospital, Joey was transferred to a nearby nursing home. He had excellent insurance coverage through his Postal Union but we made sure each and every aspect of his treatment was covered by the carrier. There are many good people in the medical field but I found out that you still had to be a strong advocate. Many of these good people are overwhelmed with their work load. There were times when "raging" was the only way to get attention. At other times, a careful "stroking" was needed. One thing is for sure, an elderly patient needs someone to aid them when they are sick. While I was feeling good and enjoying Carl's company in life, Joey's sickness was definitely stressful. I stuck religiously to my diet and exercise.

Joey's stay at the nursing home was a disaster. He suffered from "sunset syndrome" where he would have wild dreams at night. During many of these episodes, he would pull out his feeding tube. The tube was disturbing to Joey for two reasons: it felt unnatural and it hurt him when food entered his stomach. As a result, when he was suffering from nightmares, his impulse was to get rid of the tube. The nursing home was severely understaffed with qualified personnel. We would often visit Joey and find him in bed, half clothed. Considering the fact that Joey's insurance was paying nearly 300 dollars a day for his stay, it was upsetting. However, there wasn't too much we could do about it. You are truly at the mercy of the caregivers and they know it.

Each time Joey pulled his tube out of his stomach, he had to be returned to the hospital for its replacement. Joey hated the constant transfer and hated the feeding tube. He continued to lose weight. His mood was depressed. He didn't talk much but I knew he was losing the will to live. When the surgeon told me that Joey was no longer a good candidate for surgery to replace the feeding tube, I knew we were facing a difficult decision.

"Always seek out the seed of triumph in every adversity."

Og Mandino

I was really down and out by this stage of the race. I was walking down the highway that was void of any spectators. My fellow runners looked worse than I did and that was not encouraging. This was no fun and I wondered why the hell I even contemplated running this damn race. I needed a long bath, a steak and a very soft bed. I had been running for over five hours by now and was completely wasted. Emotionally, I was feeling very sorry for myself. My mind once again returned the plight of poor Joey.

The surgeon explained to both Carl and me that Joey was "failing." He elaborated that Joey's quality of life might never return and that his body was slowly deteriorating. If he replaced the feeding tube, Joey might die on the operating table. If he didn't, the tube was not working anyhow. Joey would, most likely, lose more weight. The surgeon was very honest and candid. He did not recommend the surgery. It would mean that Joey would come home to die of starvation. I cried myself to sleep that night.

The next day I knew I had to be strong for Joey. Carl and I went to the hospital and explained the options to Joey. He simply hunched up his shoulders and said: "I want to go home." He even smiled when he said it. I could barely hide my emotion. I think it may have been the saddest day of my life. I could tell in Joey's eyes that it was the right decision. Joey wanted to come back to his home to die.

We fixed up Joey's bedroom in his house with a special hospital bed and a big television. My two dogs visited him for the first time in months and jumped up on the bed. Joey laughed so hard. I loved to see him happy at home. That night, however, he had another "sunset syndrome" episode. He ranted and raved and then soiled his bed. The ever compassionate Carl changed the bed clothes and settled him down with a sedative. Joey fell into a deep sleep.

I remember earlier that night, saying good night to Joey and kissing him on the cheek. He had just watched me hug Carl good-night and it brought a smile to his face. It was the last time we looked in each other's eyes. This last look is something I will never forget. His eyes said "thank you" to me and I broke down. After his tirade later that night, he was given morphine drops to ease any pain or discomfort. He had stopped eating altogether and never really regained any type of consciousness. He slept constantly.

Joey passed away quietly on February 5th, 2006, in the early morning hours. Curiously, it was Carl's birthday. The funeral was simple and well attended by Joey's many friends and mine. Father Terry, a young priest at the Cathedral, performed the service and I gave a tearful eulogy. Carl, always the articulate attorney, gave a fine tribute to his good friend. Father Terry had gotten to know Joey in the hospital and found out about how Carl and I got back together. He confirmed our belief that it was more than coincidence that Carl and I had come together to be with Joey at the end. The priest believed that Carl had come into my life to take care of Joey and me. I also think we came into Carl's life for a reason as well.

I still recall Carl's comment when we sat with Father Terry after the service: "I am not very religious, Father," he said, "but there are really too many coincidences in this entire scenario to be just coincidence." Father Terry, his hands folded neatly in his lap, merely smiled and said: "Don't you think God is trying to tell you something?"

The facets of my old life had changed dramatically in the past six months. My new life was taking another turn in new directions. Much to my surprise, Joey's final will and testament gave me an estate worth well over a million dollars. His final gift provided me with financial independence. It also made it possible for me to take some time off from work to help take care of my Mom and Dad as they aged and also spend time with Carl. What a blessing that has been. Knowing Joey, it was important for him to give me this gift. I truly believe his prayers brought Carl into our lives and his generous bequest now provided me the opportunity to be with my parents when they needed me most.

Joey also gave us both the gift of being there with him when he left this life. Everybody kept telling us both how much we did for Joey. It became almost embarrassing. But, Joey's passing held gifts for both Carl and me. He was a special person and he left this earth in a very peaceful and proud way. He taught me how to be strong without being tough. He taught me how to love with just your eyes. Many of us think that taking care of a dying person is a burden. But there are so many things we can learn from people that are facing death. It was really my honor to be there for Joey at the end and share his final days. I am sure his spirit lives on and every time I throw out a handful of peanuts to his newly adopted squirrels in my backyard, I think of him.

Carl and I dedicated a bench to Joey at the local golf course. Now if you sit on the 13th tee at Longshore Golf Course you will see a bronze plague imprinted with the simple statement: Joey Karmanosky A Good Guy.

"Sex alleviates tension. Love causes it."

Woody Allen

I could barely see the finish line as the barren area continued. I am not usually a complainer (all those Marine roots and all) but this was one time I was really glad I had a runner partner. Much can be said for training and running a marathon with another person. They can pick you up if they can keep up. In this case, I was running with my lover and an experienced marathon runner. After his efforts to make me run over these past two miles had failed, he had enough. "We are not walking into the finish line, no way! You are going to finish this race with your head up or you will remember it forever." And so we started running. Yes, everything hurt and I remained tired, but I began to run. It is amazing what your body can do. It is truly mind over matter when it comes to moving when you are exhausted. I think I will recall this last mile more than any of the others twenty six for I found something very deep down to boost me forward. It was a good feeling. I was strong. I had to thank my running buddy for that revelation.

I was scared to hell about entering into an intimate relationship with Carl when I was closing in on my 58th birthday. I was feeling some inhibitions, both physical and emotional, I had let build up over the years. I had a new body, unknown to me as well as to anybody else. I was experiencing feelings which had been pretty much dormant for many a year.

My experience with men, looking back, may have not been the best. My college sweetheart became my brief husband. It was a marriage that may have been doomed from the beginning because it was consummated for the wrong reasons. My ex-husband felt that he had let me down when I was raped. His heritage and chauvinistic nature led to a protectiveness that was very sweet but something I did not think I needed or wanted at the time. I was a college graduate working in a new exciting arena. I felt I needed space not enclosure. I did not want to acknowledge being raped. It was not because I was ashamed. It was how I felt. It was the Miller-Marine gene. I was not brought up to waste my life pondering on negative things that for some unknown reason happened. Whether that is good or bad, I am not sure but it certainly is what I am.

As I have mentioned, there were brief interludes with some really good guys but marriage never was a serious issue. Even living together was a push. Many times I had affairs with married men. This may sound terrible but it satisfied me romantically without having to make a commitment. I liked my own space and privacy. I was hardly anti-social but I enjoyed long walks with my dogs and quiet weekends after a hectic week of work. My habit was to have a series of very social engagements followed by isolating myself at home. In recent years with my weight gain, I had not dated much. I honestly felt insecure within my own skin. The GBP surgery changed that and Carl couldn't have arrived at a better time.

While we started out well with our electronic relationship, problems developed. Carl was confident with his feeling for me but I was not sure of anything at that point. I wanted to be "friends" before committing to something else. Of course, I had used the same excuse when we first dated, decades ago. He was not pleased. I also was not very confident that he would find me physically attractive. When he first called in July, I told him that I was booked until October!! He knew nothing about my surgery or my desire to lose weight before being seen by someone who knew me 38 years ago!

When we first met in person, our relationship was strained. We had a fight even before we ever saw each other!!! I am not sure what the circumstances were but Carl has a unique sense of humor. Let's just say it is an acquired taste. He can be bluntly honest and very confident in print. He is much more caring and sincere in person. At the outset, therefore, it was a relationship of convenience. Carl needed a place to stay while he commuted to New York City on weekends and I needed someone to help with Joey.

Several weeks into our reunion, we took a long walk with the dogs on the beach. We talked about everything including some very intimate details of both our pasts. After a long marriage gone sour, Carl was hardly looking for a committed relationship. This was fine with me. But there was a certain chemistry between us and we shared common interests. We loved sports, liked to have fun and really shared a deep-seated compassion for others. Money was great but it did not define our lives. I think I really started to fall in love with him on that walk.

Being heavy does have its advantages. I had many good friends who were guys. We watched football games together and hung out socially. The factor of being attractive to each other was often taken out of the equation. I could be myself this way and let down my guard. So I did have a lot of "friends." I didn't really think I needed more so I was satisfied with this existence. It wasn't until Carl came along that I realized what I had been missing.

The first time Carl and I were intimate, we began to kiss and "make out" on my den sofa. My two black Labrador dogs, named "Ben" and "Annie," lay on the next sofa, sound asleep. Ben has always been my protector. As Carl and I continued to kiss, we both looked up to see Ben sitting a foot away from us staring right into Carl's eyes! We eventually found refuge at Joey's house, now up for sale, hearing Ben's muffled howls from across the driveway as we made love. It was so very romantic!!

I can tell you that sex gets better as you get older! We were much more experienced and knew what turned each other on. With Carl, I could communicate these needs and desires. I thought I would be embarrassed about my aging body with him but I wasn't. My breasts had definitely fallen prey to gravity and the quick loss of weight had left some excess skin around my thighs. I still remain shy about my body. I have been that way all of my life. But I bought some sexy underwear, including a black garter belt with stockings, and well . . . it was fun. Our Sundays became sex marathons and trust me, I was ready for it.

After I sold Joey's house, Carl moved in with me. Before that, Carl and I would spend the evening together and he would head back across the driveway to Joey's house to sleep. Carl liked his own time to write or read by himself. So the move-in was a test. We decided to stay in separate bedrooms. For one reason, Ben slept with me and snored like a drunken sailor. And second, we lived by different clocks. I was a morning person, rising before five a.m. to walk the dogs and go to my "spinning" class. I also love that time by myself. Carl liked to write at night and took a nap every afternoon to allow him the solitude of the night. Sometimes we would actually pass each other as I was waking and he was going to bed. In many ways, it allowed us both our individual privacy while spending a lot of time together.

Yet, still, sharing a house together with a man can be different and difficult if you are not used to it. Carl was very neat but I was set in my ways. I liked things a certain way and he admitted to be somewhat of a control freak. We really have never gone head to head in a verbal fight. That is not my style. What we have found, however, is that we can communicate any disagreements through daily emails. We email each other every day. Often times we divulge hurt feelings or problems we may be having between ourselves. Using this medium, it avoids any built up hostility that often erupts in many relationships. These emails allow us both to speak our minds and avoid long term resentments.

Carl also became my best friend. We are both very good listeners but also like to talk. With him, I have been able to share things that I have never spoken about with other people. I have some really good close girlfriends but could not share aspects of my life that I have been able to with Carl. This has really been a revelation to me. In the past I kept many things pent up inside. It is very reassuring to be able to confide and trust sharing your innermost feelings with another individual. It has helped me grow to where I really enjoy myself. Not only because I feel loved but because my ideas and feelings are important. I no longer feel judged. I feel free to share my inner self.

Early on in our relationship, I confided in Carl about my surgery. He was very sympathetic and interested in my previous life and the particulars of the operation. He would often cook dinner for me and remind me to slow down by putting up one of his fists, indicating on how big my stomach was now. He really became my biggest cheerleader. If I had any doubts about the acceptability of the surgery, it was put to rest by Carl. He was a fitness guy, too. He had run some fifteen marathons in his 25 years of running. He was in good shape. On a cold February evening, just after Joey had died, we made a bet that would continue my journey of recovery and new adventures.

MILE **26**

"It ain't over until it is over."

Yogi Berra

The Iwo Jima Monument is where the finish line was and it could be seen in foreground. The crowds had returned in huge numbers. The last mile was electric and for some reason, my aches and pains had disappeared. Isn't it amazing how your body can change with a new attitude? As I cruised at a good pace for the last mile, I could not help but think how all this started.

Within a year after I had set out my goals in that boring real estate seminar, I lost nearly 110 pounds. My goal was thirty more pounds. With Joey being so sick, I had no time to spin. I missed it but I was still losing weight through good eating and Joey, at that time, was, of course, my priority. But now Joey was gone and life needed to go on.

As I remember it, the conversation with Carl went something like this:

"I have always wanted to run a marathon," I said.

"Why don't you?" Carl asked.
"Oh, I am not sure I am ready," I responded.
"I will make it interesting. I will bet you can't!"
"How much?" I asked.
"Five bucks."
"You are on."

And so it began. Despite the cold weather, we drove up to the nearby high school track and started to run. After half way around the track, my feet were killing me and I thought I was having a heart attack. My chest ached. We stopped running.

If you are unfamiliar with a marathon or its training, it usually takes several years of running to prepare for the agonizing 26.2 mile race. It was Carl's proposal that we train and run the Marine Corps Marathon in Washington, D.C. that was in October. Considering my background, it was an obvious choice. But it was only 8 months away! After my first short run, I thought there was no way I could run that far. Carl assured me that I could go the distance or lose the bet!

We started slowly. I got up to a mile fairly quickly. We ran every other day and ran "long" every Sunday. The training was designed to keep me rested in between runs and slowly build up my endurance. Carl was an experienced marathon runner and an excellent trainer. I should add that we didn't run very fast. I was still carrying some extra pounds and I found that I didn't really enjoy running fast. It hurt! So we went slowly: 13 minute miles. We would walk some but tried to run as much as physically possible.

By spring, I was enjoying my runs and my weight was really down. I was starting to look like a runner. I loved it. Some people think that you are thin because you run or you run because you want to be thin. I am here to tell you that neither is true. You run because you like to run. You learn to run through the pain. It is sometimes hard work but more times than not, it is fun and makes you feel so alive!

We had to watch my food intake. I was burning off many calories running. It is estimated you run off about 100 calories a mile and I was up to 15 or 20 miles a week by now. We scheduled my meals to add some more calories. I was worried about stretching out my stomach but I felt confident that if I added calories through protein shakes and the like, I was fine. I also visited Doctor Floch before I had started training and he gave me the "thumbs up" on the marathon. I also cut back on my spinning and did some weights to firm up my upper body. Running uses every muscle in your body except your core-stomach area. So I did some Pilates and quite a few sit-up crunches. We also stretched before and after our runs.

It is much easier to train with someone else. Carl was a story teller and often times when I was hurting on our runs, I would just say: "Tell me a story." He would then go off on a wild soliloquy about something that happened in his past and it would take my mind of my pain. There is definitely HURT involved in this endeavor. I will not lie to you. It does hurt! But there is also a very conscious "runner's high." This is when you just feel as if you are running on cloud nine. You don't feel that you are breathing hard or working at pushing yourself. It is a very relaxing and enjoyable time. Many times, however, it does not last very long. For me, it would kick in at mile six or so in a long run, but by mile 10, I was hurting. It was nice while it lasted. There is also the feeling of being alive when you run. It sounds so simple but when your heart is pounding, your body is moving and it is a beautiful day, you feel so very much in sync with life. Running is very much a symptom of inner peace.

We made it through most of warm summer by running early. The heat affected me and I didn't enjoy it. To keep my focus, we entered a half marathon race in a nearby town. I did quite well although I was still running pretty slowly. My feet hurt so badly the last two miles I thought I was not going to make it. My business partner and good friend, Jim, was waiting for me at the finish line so I was definitely motivated to finish. I made it in just over two hours!!

Gradually, we got up to 15 and then 16 miles on our Sunday run. I was feeling comfortable in the training. I can not say it was fun but I liked the challenge. I also liked what it was doing to my body. I was down to 145 pounds. I had lost over 130 pounds and was within ten pounds of my weight in high school.

In the early fall, I got hurt. My shins hurt like hell. I could barely walk, let alone run. Carl was supportive and we iced down my legs, day and night. I needed time off to recover but time was something I did not have. The marathon was in late October, six weeks away. I went to my naturopathic doctor, "Doc" John," for help. He was an endurance athlete himself and he immediately started a series of acupuncture on my shins. I suffered from "shin splints", a common ailment among runners. It turns out I needed some new running shoes badly. The cushioning on your shoes goes quickly and after 50 miles running on them, 85% of the support is gone. Many runners rotate several pairs of shoes to avoid this happening so I was learning the hard way. The acupuncture saved me however. What normally would take months to heal, took only several weeks. Everyone, including Carl, was amazed. We ran 20 miles in early October and then began to taper off the amount of miles per week. I was ready for the marathon!

The Finish

"When I was finished, I wasn't sure I was happy because I achieved my goal or that I wouldn't ever have to do it again."

Mark Twain

The final hill was like a mountain to the finish line. Marines lined the narrow passageway to keep the thousands of screaming spectators at bay. It was the most exhilarating experience I have ever lived. All my dreams and goals had all come true. I passed under the finish line and the Marine corporal placed the medal around my neck. I gave Carl a big hug and I was done. This long journey was complete! What a trip!

I sat under the shade of some ash trees in the finishing area and lay back looking at the sky. I was exhausted but so happy. I thought of how far I really had come in the past year. It was amazing. Life had become so special and I loved every minute of it. And for the very first time in my life, I realized that I could accomplish anything!!! I was truly amazing!!!

Post Race Life

Some two years after that momentous day finishing the Marine Corps Marathon, I remain much in love with my life. My weight is still the same as the day I ran that 26.2 miles and Carl is still very much part of my existence. I am healthy, energetic and happy. I have reached every one of my goals that I wrote that day in 2005. This accomplishment makes me feel wonderful. However, the memories of the journey of my transformation may be more important to me than the goals themselves.

There have been some huge changes and some tears shed since that marathon day. I have lost both my parents in a six month period. My father died of cancer after a courageous but painful fight. Five months later, my mother woke in the middle of the night and told her caregiver: "Dad is here. It is time for me to go." She then promptly stopped breathing. Their absence is still very much with me. I shall miss them forever.

The country I love as well has taken a different turn and I find my career threatened by a housing crisis. As this nation gears up for change under a new dynamic administration, I wonder how these changes will affect my life? At my age, it is somewhat scary. But change is good at any age. I learned that when I chose to have the GBP. To hold on to the past is not healthy. There are always new adventures. You just have to keep looking for them.

I continue to run, spin and swim. I have fallen in love with golf. I find myself less of a spectator than a participant now. It is far more fulfilling. I work less, play harder. I still love to laugh and do it more often. My ten symptoms of inner peace remain by my computer. I say them constantly.

Most of my good friends are still my good friends.

I have new neighbors in a bigger house with loving hearts like Joey. He would like them. I have traveled to exotic islands, toured New England in an RV and skied the slopes of Vail. My dogs still wake me up early in the morning, Ben still snores and Carl still makes my heart flutter.

Most important, the marathon of change that transformed me is still happening each and every day of my life!!!

Jo Ann Miller
Basye, Virginia
September 2009

Acknowledgements

This book would have not been possible without the expert oversight of Addison Fletcher, my intellectual soul mate. He came up with the idea when I showed him my 2005 diary. He put me to work and encouraged me every step of the way. Also to Dr. Craig Floch and his staff at Fairfield County Bariatrics & Surgical Specialists. He is a wonderful surgeon and a great guy. To my "readers": Debbie Wood, Cindy Harper (twice), Tom Allen, Nonnie Thompson, Rita Lazzeroni, Carol Johnson (who didn't like it at first reading which caused me to work harder!), Jayne Hynes, Lucy Hixon and Louise Craft, who edited it on her summer holiday! A special thanks to "Uncle Johnny," my hero, for the Foreword and the wind beneath his wings, "Aunt Annie." Thank you to Dr. Hochstrasser for permission to use her expertise. Thank you to all. You are very dear to my heart.

www.ingramcontent.com/pod-product-compliance
Lightning Source LLC
Chambersburg PA
CBHW020246290526
45784CB00003B/1123

* 9 7 8 1 4 3 2 7 5 5 0 5 8 *